# DETERMINED

*Dedicated to "E-N" and "I-N."*
*Kristen, without your love and support, this dream of mine would not have been possible. You are my rock and my much better half. Thank you for constantly pointing me to the cross.*
*Kristin, your accountability, structure, and encouragement have made all the difference at The Physician Philosopher. I couldn't imagine running this business with anyone else.*

*Note: Any client names and stories in this book have been altered in order to protect client privacy (except Paul's name because he is a living legend). However, the salient points and details of their stories remain intact.*

# DETERMINED

HOW BURNED OUT DOCTORS CAN THRIVE
IN A BROKEN MEDICAL SYSTEM

JAMES D. TURNER, MD

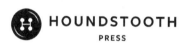

HOUNDSTOOTH
PRESS

DETERMINED
*How Burned Out Doctors Can Thrive in a Broken Medical System*

ISBN   HARDCOVER: 978-1-5445-3150-2
      PAPERBACK: 978-1-5445-3149-6
      EBOOK: 978-1-5445-3148-9

# CONTENTS

# INTRODUCTION

FROM HIS JAIL cell, he could see the blue skies. And the horizon. That was about the only redeeming feature about Robben Island. His cell was eight feet by seven feet and contained no plumbing. It was constantly damp. This is where he lived at night. During the day, he worked on the limestone, which would permanently damage his eyesight from the glaring sun. It was in the Robben Island Prison that he spent eighteen of his twenty-seven years in jail as a political prisoner. He would acquire tuberculosis and was not allowed regular outside correspondence except once every six months. While imprisoned, he wasn't even allowed to attend his son's funeral when his son died in a car crash in 1969. He was physically and emotionally abused during his imprisonment. Why? Because he believed he deserved equal rights as a Black man in South Africa during apartheid.

While his physical and emotional health may have suffered, Nelson Mandela's spirit was strong. He refused to bow to his captors. They could take his clothes. They could force him to work. They could emotionally and physically abuse him. Yet, Mandela recognized that his mind was the one thing that he—and he alone—could control. He refused to be the victim in a situation that would see most people crumble. Mandela refused to give up control of what mattered most—his will.

Nelson Mandela continued to study. He taught others what he learned. Throughout his imprisonment, he remained singularly focused on his anti-apartheid mission. After twenty-seven years as a political prisoner, Nelson Mandela was released in 1990. He then led negotiations with the African National Congress to end apartheid. Three years later, he was awarded the Nobel Peace Prize. And in 1994, over twenty million South Africans turned out to cast ballots in the first-ever multiracial elections. Nelson Mandela won an overwhelming majority of the votes on his way to becoming the first-ever non-white president of South Africa, a position he held from 1994 until 1999.

For most, becoming the victim of a bad situation is all too easy. We let our tormentors control much more than our emotional and physical wellness. We also relinquish control over our minds. We cease to be autonomous beings. What Nelson Mandela realized is that it is our God-given right to *choose* how we see our reality.

We saw this in the now infamous Stanford prison experiment where the students were randomly selected to either be a jailer or prisoner in a role-playing scenario. After a very short period of time, the jailers started to abuse the prisoners. In turn, the prisoners started to assume a victim mentality. That is how they saw their reality. Even though it was just a role-playing experiment, it had to be stopped due to the harm the jailers caused to the prisoners.

Yet, Mandela didn't allow his captors to control his mind or the perspective, paradigm, or narrative his mind produced. Even in a real-life prison environment, Mandela continued his agenda of ending racism on all accounts in order to have a multiracial South Africa that was at peace. As he left prison, Mandela recounted, "As I walked out the door toward the gate that would lead to my freedom, I knew if I didn't leave my bitterness and hatred behind, I'd still be in prison." How was Mandela able to do this in a real prison situation when the Stanford prisoners in the experiment could not? It is all about perspective.

## THERE IS NO "THERE" THERE

We were standing in the fairway on the second hole of the West golf course at the Bermuda Run Country Club when it happened. My friend Mike and I were getting out to play a quick nine holes with the hopes of taking a break from our busy work lives and watching our kids. I was also trying to escape my raging case of burnout. Unfortunately, that's not what happened.

It started that morning. I had been taking a prescription medication called propranolol since being diagnosed with an essential tremor—a neurology resident had noticed the tremor while I was performing a lumbar puncture as a third-year medical student. As I went to open the bottle, I realized I had forgotten to refill my prescription. I fulfilled the truism that "doctors make the worst patients." *No big deal*, I thought, *I'll fill my propranolol later. I'll be playing golf. This will be a super low-key day. Who cares if my hands shake a bit? Nothing a beer or two can't fix.*

And I was right. Missing out on the propranolol wasn't a big deal. At least not at first. Mike and I were standing in the fairway on the second hole when the group behind us drove their ball from the tees. Hearing the noise, I looked back just in time to see a little white blur flying about 100 mph past my head. That's when it happened. The palpitations were sudden. My heart felt like it was in my throat. And my entire face was flushed. This was fight-or-flight in the most severe form I had ever experienced. Everything in my body told me that I was in mortal danger. I was experiencing my first panic attack.

For the uninitiated, teeing a golf ball into the group ahead while they are within reach of your drive is a big "no-no" in golf. A golf ball flying 100 mph can do much more than break a windowpane. It can also cause major trauma to anyone standing in the way. This is why you never tee off when someone is standing in the fairway. It is like firing a gun downrange and hoping that you don't connect with the person who happens to be standing in the way.

As the ball slowly rolled to a stop, my emotions went through the roof. That is when I turned to Mike and said, "I'm going to need you to handle this when they come down here. I can't control my emotions right now."

I am an otherwise cool, calm, and collected kind of guy. Particularly in stressful situations. This serves me well in medicine because it turns out that no one likes an anesthesiologist who cannot keep their cool when the shit hits the fan. So, when my body went into DEFCON 1 due to a tiny, white, circular object that didn't even hit me, I knew immediately something was wrong.

## IT IS ALL JUST STRESS, RIGHT?

Let's back up a bit and put this all into perspective. Then we can zoom back in on my journey through burnout to connect the dots, and how that led to my experience on the second hole of the Bermuda Run golf course.

When I first became a coach for burned-out physicians, someone pointed me to a personality test called the Enneagram. While controversy exists over the validity of the Enneagram, I personally found it helpful. After taking the test, it told me that I was a Type 3, Wing 2 on the Enneagram—what is known as an "Achiever" or "Charmer." I learned that my life is about productivity and accomplishments. In other words, I need to achieve in order to be happy.

Type 3 personalities tend to be self-assured, confident, and driven by ambition. We are the sort of people that are commonly asked, "How do you get everything done?" Type 3s care very much about what other people think, which proves problematic since our self-worth comes from accomplishments, accolades, and achievements.

After taking the test, it didn't take long for me to see this insatiable appetite for achievement in my own life. In college, I was named the E.B. Kennedy scholar after winning one of two full-ride scholarships offered by Erskine College following a rigorous, multiday in-person interview process involving hundreds of high school students. While in medical school at Wake Forest, I was elected the class president and then student body president. And, during residency, I was elected one of two chief residents.

After training, I was earning half a million dollars a year, winning teaching awards in record fashion, and publishing multiple peer-reviewed, randomized control trials in my first year as an attending. I was also running a successful six-figure business. I was the host of two five-star podcasts (*The Physician Philosopher* and *Money Meets Medicine*, which I previously hosted with my friend Ryan Inman) and even authored a successful book teaching personal finance to physicians. My teaching evaluations were stellar, and I was a pretty good clinician, too.

I checked every box of a Type 3 Enneagram. I won the big awards along with every democratically elected position during my medical training. On the outside, I looked like I had it all figured out. Yet, if I am being honest, I was also entirely burned out and frankly quite miserable on the inside.

With everything I had accomplished, I wondered why I wasn't happier at the end of my journey. After all those long hours and sleepless nights in training to become a physician, was this really it? Without many answers, I began to self-medicate. I didn't self-medicate with cocaine, heroin, ecstasy, LSD, or marijuana. Instead, I self-medicated through my addiction to what is known as an arrival fallacy, a term coined by Tal Ben-Shahar—a Harvard-trained psychologist. Tal Ben-Shahar described the arrival fallacy phenomenon in an article in the *New York Times* as an "illusion that once we make it, once we attain our goal or reach our destination, we will reach lasting happiness."[1]

---

1   A.C. Shilton, "You Accomplished Something Great. So Now What?," The New York Times, May 28, 2019, https://www.nytimes.com/2019/05/28/ smarter-living/you-accomplished-something-great-so-now-what.html.

If you aren't sure whether or not you have ever succumbed to an arrival fallacy, tell me if this sounds familiar. Do you remember feeling that when you got to residency, things would be better than medical school, only to find that you were burned out in residency? Did you think that the burnout of residency would surely get better when you became an attending physician making a physician income? When that didn't work, did you think that getting promoted to partner or advancing in the academic ranks might improve your situation?

For those of us who suffer from an arrival fallacy, each time we accomplish something new, it brings a jolt of short-lived satisfaction. Unfortunately, it never seems to last. So, our desire to solve our dissatisfaction continues. From this place, you may have decided to buy the doctor house, a nicer car, expensive gadgets and gizmos, designer clothes and handbags, or a dream vacation. All of these purchases were an attempt to find the sustained happiness that seemed to elude you. Like me, you likely found that any happiness you experienced was fleeting. The pot of gold you hoped to find at the end of the rainbow wasn't where you thought it would be. The promised land wasn't so promising after all.

If you have ever looked for happiness in any of these things and found that life in medicine wasn't all that it was chalked up to be, you likely suffer from an arrival fallacy, too. This is called a fallacy for a reason. It isn't true. It turns out that Gertrude Stein had it right when she said, "There is no 'there' there." With less and less autonomy over what time I would get home, not feeling like I belonged either as a member of the team or attached to a deeper sense of purpose at the hospital, and having the typical imposter syndrome that plagues many physicians...I was burning out fast, and my arrival fallacies were the only thing that kept my head above the water. There is a problem with this routine, though. It isn't a long-term solution.

Once we arrive, the accomplishments, achievements, and purchases lead to a short-lived hit of dopamine without the long-term, sustained satisfaction we want. It is a bit like doing high-speed intervals on a hedonic treadmill. While running each interval as fast as we can, we get short reprieves for our efforts when we finish our interval, only to be forced to go back onto the never-ending treadmill shortly thereafter for the next sprint. Quickly, I found out that short-term happiness and long-term fulfillment are not the same. All of my accomplishments were a drug I had become dependent on to keep me from drowning from stress and burnout. When burnout came knocking only a couple of years into my career as an attending physician, I became dependent on the arrival fallacy to escape. I was an arrival fallacy junkie.

Then, one day, the supply of arrivals dried up. The accomplishments weren't coming as quickly. Buying the doctor house didn't help, nor did the naturally aspirated, V8 powered manual transmission sedan that I bought (*but it did sound great!*). With an addiction to accomplishment, and my self-worth and fulfillment being attached to it, it didn't take long for me to start drowning when four (*yes, as in the number after three*) Assistant Program Director (APD) positions opened up, and I wasn't chosen for any of them despite being qualified for the job and expressing interest. While I found out later that I had been considered for the APD role, the fact was that four other people were appointed by departmental leadership, including two of my best friends from my residency class. The four new APDs were all incredible people, yet to say this stung would be a massive understatement. For years, being a leader in the residency program was the direction I thought my career had been heading, and the door had been slammed in my face. Not once, but *four times*.

When my chain of "arrivals" finally broke in a harsh and sudden way, my demons came out. I was in arrival fallacy withdrawal. My professional autonomy over my career had been stripped from me. And I certainly didn't feel appreciated. I was burning out, and I was starting to have symptoms from it. Or so I thought. First, there were the headaches. Then my essential tremor started getting worse. Every room felt like a sauna. My wife, Kristen, and I were also getting into a lot of heated arguments, which was new for us. I started to resent my job. I wasn't sleeping. In fact, I realized that I hadn't slept through the night for more than ten to twenty days in the previous twelve months. Each night, I'd wake up three or four times, amped up and unable to fall back to sleep.

Some of my friends and family thought it was because I had too much on my plate. *It turned out this was one of the reasons that I wasn't chosen for the four APD positions—in addition to my proclivity for strong opinions about taboo topics like personal finance and burnout.* Yet, I had always managed to juggle all of the balls in the air without much difficulty. In the end, something else was going on, which takes us back to the panic attack I experienced on the second hole of the Bermuda Run golf course that fateful day when I ran out of propranolol.

After that little white golf ball took hold of my emotions, I went to my family medicine doctor to put it all together. Fortunately, she knew her stuff. The TSH she ordered ended up being undetectable (<0.1 mU/ml). A few weeks later, my endocrinologist diagnosed me with Graves' disease. At the time, I wasn't sure if my Graves' disease had led to my burnout, or if my burnout was uncovered more easily because of my autoimmune disease. Was it the chicken or the egg? At this point, I believe it was the latter. And I'm not alone in that theory.

In a 2018 observational study published in *JAMA*,[2] Dr. Song and colleagues took 100,000 individuals who had stress or stress-related disorders and matched them with over one million individuals without stress or stress-related disorders. They compared the data to more than 125,000 siblings of the cohort who had not experi-

---

2    Huan Song, Fang Fang, Gunnar Tomasson, et al., "Association of Stress-Related Disorders With Subsequent Autoimmune Disease," JAMA 319 no. 23 (2018): 2388–2400, https://doi.org/10.1001/jama.2018.7028.

enced stress or stress-related disorders as well. The question they were seeking to answer was whether someone who experienced continual stress was more or less likely to develop autoimmune disorders, like Graves' disease. What they found is that patients with stress or stress-related disorders had much higher rates of autoimmune diseases, including specifically thyroid disease.

Was the stress from my burnout associated with the Graves' disease or vice versa? In my experiment of N=1, I came to a conclusion similar to Dr. Song's after starting my methimazole. With treatment, my symptoms improved. My labs showed that I was euthyroid, too. However, despite treatment, my burnout didn't get better, and neither did my arrival fallacy addiction. In fact, they both got worse. I didn't feel like I had professional autonomy. The prior career path I'd been traveling to become an APD was at its end. I started having some trouble with imposter syndrome, too. *Maybe I just wasn't good enough to be a leader in my department?*

My personal autonomy was also under attack as I had little control over my time and when I got home each day. My life felt controlled by a constantly growing to-do list, and I only felt temporarily better when I accomplished more. Yet, there were never enough hours in the day to accomplish everything that I needed to get done in order for my arrival fallacy to keep me afloat. As a husband, father, physician, and entrepreneur, I had a hard time keeping up. Even when I'd have a momentary hit of dopamine from an accomplishment, it was short-lived. I was suffering from all of the symptoms of burnout.

That's when the anxiety and depression accompanying my burnout became very real for me. As I started to go down, my primary care physician threw me a life preserver called escitalopram and therapy. This made things better for a bit, but my life outside the public eye was still a train wreck. I felt burned out and completely out of balance. Scarier still, I felt like I didn't belong despite being surrounded by people who loved me. While the escitalopram, therapy, and becoming euthyroid were all helpful, none of these modalities cured my burnout. Instead, what helped reduce my burnout was something that I was *much* more skeptical about as a burned-out physician—shifting my perspective through coaching. It was because of this skepticism that I initially ignored people's advice to try physician coaching.

When I finally decided to try it, coaching would change my life. Eventually, this led me to spend the time and money to become a certified coach myself and to start a physician-only coaching program called the Alpha Coaching Experience, or ACE as the cool kids call it, where we have helped hundreds of doctors defeat their burnout and create a life they love. It is because of this work that I wrote this book—to teach you the concepts we teach our clients in ACE. I fought against coaching for a long time, and as I write this, I realize you may have the same skepticism I once had.

After all, the burnout I was experiencing wasn't my fault, right? It was the broken medical system that was causing my problem. Like many physicians, I felt that I was the victim of burnout, not the cause of it. In fact, I remember people asking me about this in multiple interviews early in the life of *The Physician Philosopher,* and telling them that I thought "blaming the victim" of burnout was a baseless and harmful exercise. It was the system that needed to be fixed. Not the doctor. So, if it wasn't *me* that needed to change, surely changing my external circumstances was the best course of action. At least, that's what I thought.

## CHANGING CIRCUMSTANCES

When facing burnout, most physicians think about making a change. They take a new job, go part-time, or think about starting a side gig to make more nonclinical income. This is usually done in an attempt to free themselves from their current situation. A 2020 survey of over 1,200 physicians performed by MDLinx showed that 48% of physician respondents were considering a career change.[3] This included 34% of doctors who were considering a change in their practice and 26% who said they were considering retiring, leaving patient care, closing their practice, or quitting medicine to start a new career. By changing their circumstances, these doctors think it will end their suffering. If they can't do that, the least they can do is escape their bad situation for a little while by working somewhere else.

It doesn't always work, though. Think about it. Do all doctors who change jobs find the happiness and fulfillment they currently want? Nope. Not even close. In fact, one survey performed by an Atlanta-based recruiting agency found that over 50% of doctors will leave their first job within three to five years after training. This is despite telling everyone it was a "great job" when they found it. It isn't just new doctors that think about changing jobs or leaving medicine either. According to an article in the *Washington Post*, after the pandemic hit, 30% of physicians considered joining The Great Resignation and leaving medicine altogether.[4] Despite these changes, it is common for a physician to change jobs and to end up being just as burned out six months after taking the new job. This is what happens when burned-out doctors don't spend the time determining what the actual cause of their burnout is before making the change. When we change jobs without doing the necessary thought work, we are treating the symptom. Not the disease.

---

3    John Murphy, "Nearly Half of Doctors are Rethinking Their Careers, Finds COVID-19 Survey," MDLinx, November 6, 2020, https://www.mdlinx.com/article/nearly-half-of-doctors-are-rethinking-their-careers-finds-covid-19-survey/32iphKz3vp3DlR3LuXOBkA.
4    William Wan, "Burned out by the Pandemic, 3 in 10 Health-Care Workers Consider Leaving the Profession: After a Year of Trauma, Doctors, Nurses and Other Health Workers are Struggling to Cope," The Washington Post, April 22, 2021, https://www.washingtonpost.com/health/2021/04/22/health-workers-covid-quit/.

As a coaching client, I learned to do the thought work before changing circumstances. That's why I spend the first half of this book describing the problem and our need to master our mindset first. Like in medicine, it is necessary to make the diagnosis before we can determine a successful treatment plan. In addition to that, when it comes to burnout, the thought work is often sufficient in and of itself to allow doctors to fall back in love with medicine without having to change jobs at all. When we put in the thought work, it can empower us to be able to deal with any and every situation, no matter how bad.

Evident in Nelson Mandela's story, and the teachings of many stoic philosophers, is the idea that external situations may be out of our control. Many stop at this realization and then wallow in self-pity. After realizing that sometimes there is nothing they can do about things outside their control, all hope seems lost. It doesn't have to be this way, though.

We do not have to let external circumstances stop us in our tracks. And, odds are that if you are reading this book, then you aren't going to stop there, either. Why? Because you are likely sick and tired of being sick and tired. You are a brave and courageous physician. You are looking for a different way to view the problems in your life, including the burnout that is wreaking havoc in your soul. You aren't going to give up that easily. If you are reading this book, you recognize that while we cannot control our external circumstances there is one thing we can always control: our focus.

## NOT ALL PRISONERS ARE IN PRISON

Mandela taught us that we can work to change a broken system (apartheid, in his situation) while we simultaneously refuse to be broken ourselves. Said differently, you can fix a broken system while you *simultaneously* refuse to let it control you. How we react is determined by our perspectives, paradigms, and narratives.

Like Mandela, doctors may not be able to control the circumstances and situations around us in medicine. We cannot control the broken nature of the electronic medical record (EMR) system. Or the well-meaning yet intolerable administrators who buy us coffee thinking that a little caffeine is going to solve our burnout. Doctors cannot stop the constant micromanagement insurance companies cause that prevents us from caring for our patients. Despite this, we don't have to let the broken system control *us*. We can rage against this broken machine (*because medicine IS broken*) while we simultaneously control our internal response. The administrators and insurance companies can see us as a cog in the wheel of this machine or just a number on a balance sheet. Yet, it is up to us to control who we are and what we do when tough situations arise.

The point is this: we have two choices when faced with external circumstances that we see as unfair or unjust. The first choice is that we can do what most do and choose to label ourselves as a victim of a bad situation or circumstance. We can wallow in the defeat and misery caused by a broken medical system. We can bide our time until the system magically changes or until we are able to retire. Or we can choose to be the hero in a broken situation.

## VICTIM OR HERO? THE CHOICE IS YOURS.

Do we really want to self-identify as a victim? No. We don't. And it will not lead to the change we want. How do I know? Because when I was burned out, I labeled myself as a victim, and I've seen countless other physicians do the same. There were months on end that I sat on my back porch drinking an IPA while complaining to my wife about the state of medicine. While it felt good to commiserate and to blame everything on something external, labeling myself as a victim and commiserating did not help. I wasn't able to move forward.

Think about it. Do any doctors who assume the role of victim really defeat their moral injury? No. They don't. In fact, this is exactly what the system wants: for doctors to remain silent while the insurance companies in control continue to reap the rewards. Just like the prisoners in the Stanford prison experiment who became depressed and broken down even when other study participants assumed the role of prison guards.

Like the Stanford prisoners, you can choose bitterness, anger, and defeat. You can change jobs, go part-time, or try to create the financial freedom you need to leave medicine completely. In so doing, you have positioned yourself as the bitter victim trying to break out of jail. And this, my friends, is the problem. When we choose the role of victim, we have already lost in the most important way. We have lost control of our own thoughts, feelings, and the way we show up in this world. We have chosen the way of bitterness and anger that Mandela warned us against.

There is a better way. One that provides hope instead of burnout. Like Mandela, we can choose to position ourselves as the hero of our story instead of assuming the role of the victim. Many of our physician clients come into coaching expecting the coaches to tell them how to make the changes they need in life to be happy. Maybe they think we will teach them how to chart more efficiently, make more money, or transition jobs in order to find fulfillment in medicine. That's not what happens, though. After our clients learn the skill of mastering their internal focus created by their thoughts, most of them end up doing the opposite of changing their jobs or leaving medicine. Most end up falling back in love with medicine—right where they are—without needing to change their circumstances at all.

This is why we always teach clients that—before they change jobs, go part-time, or start a physician side gig to create nonclinical income—they must first do the thought work to make the right diagnosis. They must spend the time determining the cause of their burnout. Just like we can only prescribe the best treatment for a patient when we make an accurate diagnosis, we must make decisions based on the strength of a proper mindset instead of from the scarcity created by a bad environment. As doctors, we often feel trapped in medicine by moral injury, or we feel that the reality of working in medicine hasn't lived up to the dream we hoped it would. We feel unappreciated, unheard, or overworked. We feel we have no control over the administrators and insurance companies that seem to rule our world. Yet, when we get home late for the umpteenth time, when the charting seems endless and we are overwhelmed by massive amounts of debt or non-competes in our contracts, when conflict-of-interest policies seem unfair...We. Still. Have. A. Choice.

We can realize that we are only a victim if we choose to be. We can stand firm knowing that we are strong, smart, intelligent, resilient, and enough. Right now. Just the way that we are.

## WHAT IF THE JOURNEY IS THE DESTINATION?

Growing up, Rhett's father was a physician. He was also an alcoholic who made some poor life choices. During Rhett's adolescence, his dad decided to uproot his family and make a career transition. Rhett's father wasn't happy with his job in medicine. So, instead of doing the thought work to figure out why, he tried to escape his situation like most other burned-out doctors. In the end, the new job didn't work out for Rhett's father. That's when he looked for answers in the bottom of a bottle. Rhett's physician father lost his job, and eventually his life, after succumbing to alcoholism. That's when his family went through hard financial times. This consequential decision to change jobs was permanently imprinted on Rhett's mind when he became a physician himself.

Early in his career, Rhett discovered the Financial Independence

Retire Early, or FIRE, community. (For the uninformed, the FIRE movement is predicated on the idea that people spend much less than they earn, save the difference, and achieve financial independence very early. This has led some doctors to retire in their thirties and forties.)

With his sights set squarely on being able to achieve FIRE and leave his job in medicine, Rhett moved to a rural area of the country where the pay was well above the national average. He was making great money and great progress toward his financial goals. Yet, there was a problem. Both he and his family were unhappy outside of the big city. Nonetheless, he didn't want to make the same mistakes his father had and decided he would rather be unhappy in his job in medicine and be able to accomplish his financial goals.

Rhett stayed at his job as an intensivist because it paid well and provided the financial security that he desperately desired. That's when Rhett came into coaching to discuss his job in medicine, the marriage problems he was having because of it, and his family's overall discontent with their situation. On one call, I asked Rhett, "Why stay in a job you don't like in a small rural town where your wife cannot finish her doctoral training and that your family does not enjoy?"

The answer didn't take long. "If I stay in this job for just five more years, I will be able to hit FIRE and retire from medicine," he said. "If I move closer to the city, I will make less money and delay our financial independence." Rhett was letting his father's financial failures control his family's life. He had a victim mindset. After a series of coaching calls, Rhett came to realize that he didn't have to let his past, which he could not control, determine his future, which he *could* control.

Rhett needed thought work to reclaim his autonomy. That's when I asked him, "Rhett, would you rather be miserable working in a place and a job that you and your family don't like so that you can retire from medicine in five years...or move to a job closer to the city where you feel like you belong and take the risk that it might delay your retirement to ten years?"

What I was asking Rhett to realize was that getting to FIRE was an arrival fallacy. Getting to financial independence faster wasn't the answer to being happier. He was making himself (and his family) miserable on the journey to get there. What if he could learn to enjoy the journey such that he never wanted to make it to his destination? What if he played the infinite game instead of the finite game? What if, in fact, the journey *was* the destination?

When he thought about this, he quickly realized he would rather work in a job he actually liked in a location that was better for his family for ten years than to destroy himself in a job he hated for five years just so he could retire early. He was starting to master the autonomy, belonging, and competence of a self-determined physician. These are all topics I will cover in this book.

On our last call together, Rhett was sitting in a new BMW that he had been wanting to buy for a long time but refused to purchase because it would slow down his financial journey. Rhett started to see all the things in his life that he had been limiting, all for the sake of being able to retire as early as possible from medicine. In his new BMW 3 Series convertible, he shared the big news that after a lot of coaching and discussions with his wife, he and his family decided to move to the big city where they would be closer to friends and family, and where they felt like they belonged.

Ironically, it turned out that his assumption about earning less money in a better location didn't end up being true either. The job he found was desperately in need of his specialty. Rhett ended up with more nonclinical time *and* more money. His wife was able to take the steps she needed to finish her doctoral work, and his family and friends were nearby. In the end, he got to have his cake and eat it, too. Like Nelson Mandela, Rhett refused to be the victim of his situation while simultaneously standing up for the change he and his family needed.

## WHAT YOU'LL DISCOVER

While this book is meant to empower the individual physician who is struggling with burnout, there is also a lot of work to be done on the systemic and systematic front, which is why I will outline the problems that exist. Truthfully, until we create cultures that weed out the systematic causes of burnout in medicine outlined in the beginning of this book, the problems physicians have will continue to exist.

The good news, however, is that you can improve your individual situation in the meantime, regardless of how bad medicine may seem. If you want to continue to label yourself as a victim and wallow in your burned-out self-defeat, then this is not the book for you. However, if you want to learn how to become the hero of your story, or learn how to bite your thumb at the medical system that mistreats medical professionals, or if you are willing to transition from burned out to the badass boss of a life you love, then stick with me. You have found the book for you.

This book, then, is broken into four parts. In Part 1, we will outline the current state of medicine and the systematic problems that ail the burned-out doctor when hospitals choose to focus on profit instead of on the medical professionals on the front line. In Part 2, we will dive into the impact these systemic causes have on individual doctors. In Part 3, we will discuss the tools I teach our physician clients to defeat their individual burnout and reclaim their autonomy. And finally, in Part 4, I will provide some powerful paradigms that doctors can use while fighting in the medical arena.

So, I'll ask you. What is your story? What is holding you back from making the change that you know you need to make? Are you telling yourself that you are helpless to remedy your situation? Are you giving your autonomy to someone else? You don't have to. You are not helpless. You are strong, courageous, and brave enough to figure this out. Let me show you the way.

# PART 1

# THE PROBLEMATIC STATE OF MEDICINE

"We can't solve problems by using the same kind
of thinking we used when we created them."
—Albert Einstein

# CHAPTER 1

# Autonomy

"Because to take away a man's freedom of choice, even
his freedom to make the wrong choice, is to manipulate
him as though he were a puppet and not a person."
—Madeleine L'Engle

"NO, DADDY! I want to do it by my-own-big-girl-self!"

These are the words that assaulted my eardrums after taking out
a toothbrush, slapping some toothpaste on the bristles, and asking
my four-year-old to open her mouth. One thing was clear. Anna
Ruth didn't want my help. *And yes, Anna Ruth says "my-own-big-
girl-self" as if it is one word.*

While I thought that the terrible twos or the dreaded threenager
phase—what we called all of our three-year-olds who acted like
temperamental teenagers—were bad, it turned out the age of four
was challenging, too. With four trips around the sun, Anna Ruth
was certain about at least one thing. She didn't like other people
micromanaging her. She wanted independence and control in her
life. Even if she wasn't doing something right, she wanted the freedom to choose. While I thought I was trying to help her brush her

teeth, put her shoes on, or comb her hair, that is *not* how she saw it. To Anna Ruth, I was stripping her of her autonomy. Anna Ruth was teaching me that taking someone's ability to choose for themselves was a sure-fire way to torment someone.

None of us like being micromanaged, controlled, or otherwise coerced. We understand this from a very young age—*apparently at least by the age of four*. Worse still is when this coercion leads to bad outcomes in our life or in the lives of our patients. This is borne out in the 2021 annual Medscape *National Physician Burnout and Suicide Report*.[5]

Burnout is two times higher in physicians than in the general population. It is not just the prevalence that is alarming. The potential consequences of burnout on medical professionals are also staggering, which in burned-out individuals includes higher rates of substance and alcohol use, depression, and suicide. On the systematic front, burnout has also been linked with

- higher physician turnover;
- worse patient care and outcomes;
- decreased patient satisfaction;
- higher healthcare costs; and
- increased risk for major medical errors.[6]

Burnout is costly for physicians and for the patients under our care. It is expensive for the business of medicine as well. Current

---

5    Leslie Kane, "'Death by 1000 Cuts': Medscape National Physician Burnout & Suicide Report 2021," Medscape, January 22, 2021, https://www.medscape.com/slideshow/2021-lifestyle-burnout-6013456.

6    Daniel Tawfik et al., "Physician Burnout, Well-Being, and Work Unit Safety Grades in Relationship to Reported Medical Errors," *Mayo Clinic Proceedings* 93, no. 11 (November 2018): 1571–80, https://doi.org/10.1016/j.mayocp.2018.05.014.

estimates show that burnout costs the healthcare system approximately $5 billion per year. That's $5 billion with a "B." Some estimates are even higher. This is not surprising given that it costs a hospital approximately $250,000 to $1 million to replace a burned-out physician who decides to leave.[7] That number may seem high, but when you consider the lost revenue from physician turnover, it provides clarity. For example, when a physician leaves, so does their patient panel. The procedures on their schedule also remain unperformed. It takes months to credential a new physician and to get them up to speed. All the while, this downtime quickly adds up to lost revenue. This is one of the many reasons why it is worth it for hospital leadership to invest *at least* $7,600 per year per physician in efforts to solve the systemic problem of burnout in medicine. Why? Because at an individual level, burnout has been estimated to cost ~$7,600 per physician. Burnout is expensive!

The return on investment in such efforts would dwarf any cost. In fact, a recent intervention at the Cleveland Clinic that included a peer-based coaching and mentoring program for doctors was estimated to have saved the hospital a staggering $133 million in physician retention. So, if burnout is expensive, and investments placed toward thwarting burnout prove helpful, why isn't more being done? To answer this, let's look at the origin and complicated nature of burnout.

## IS BURNOUT THE WRONG WORD?

Before we dive into the rest of this book, let's address the elephant in the room. The word "burnout" has come under fire recently (*pun*

---

7    Shasha Han et al., "Estimating the Attributable Cost of Physician Burnout in the United States," *Annals of Internal Medicine* 170, no. 11 (June 2019): 784–90, https://doi.org/10.7326/M18-1422.

*intended*). The reason is that burnout, which was first coined by German psychologist Herbert Freudenberger in the 1970s, implies to some that the mental anguish and trauma that physicians experience is "caused by" the burned-out doctor. In other words, some feel that the term burnout blames the victim. In an ever-growing culture where victim shaming and victim blaming are on par with things like racism or sexism, you can see why this narrative is problematic.

Instead, some have suggested that we use the term "moral injury," which implies that the injury is happening *to* the physician instead of being self-inflicted *by* the physician. To the unacquainted, moral injury occurs when medical professionals have the ability, knowledge, and know-how to help a patient but are unable to do so because of systematic failures that prevent the care from happening. In other words, moral injury exists when doctors feel that the system is causing harm to their patients and colleagues, and that they are helpless to prevent it. This phenomenon causes profound moral disorientation and emotional trauma. It is also distinctly different from burnout. For this reason, I want to state one thing unequivocally in the first chapter of this book:

The causes of burnout and moral injury are systemic and systematic in nature. The causes happen *to* doctors (not because of them) just like Mandela's treatment while a political prisoner on Robben Island happened *to* Mandela (and not because of him).

The medical system is broken. To illustrate this point, we can look at the National Academy of Medicine, which brought together multiple stakeholders and constituents to form the Action Collaborative on Clinician Well-Being and Resilience. Through this effort, the collaborative identified over seventy factors that contribute to clinician well-being and resilience (*"resilience," by the way, is another naughty word among physicians because of the victim implications*). Read that again. There are over *SEVENTY* factors that impact physician well-being and, therefore, that impact the opposite—moral injury and burnout. This seventy-item model includes items such as litigation risk, reimbursement, bureaucracy, coping skills, workplace safety and culture, leadership, the electronic medical record system, and administrative responsibilities. And this is just to name a few.

What this shows us is that clinician well-being and burnout are complex and multifactorial. Medicine is a complete dumpster fire. I'm sure you don't need convincing, though. As you can imagine, this overwhelming list of more than seventy items makes it less than practical—and maybe even impossible—to determine the few items that matter most. Not to worry, however! Models have been proposed to help alleviate the multifactorial nature of burnout, like the one introduced at Penn State. Adapted from Maslow's hierarchy of needs, it's called the Health Professional Wellness Hierarchy, shown below.[8]

Shaped like a pyramid, the base of this model states that physicians must first take care of their basic physical and mental health needs before anything else can be corrected. Only then can we move on to higher needs like appreciation, respect, and the ability to contribute meaningfully. What sort of basic needs are they referring to that must first be met? Tasks that include sleeping enough, having time to breastfeed, eating well, and having access to regular bathroom breaks.

Think about that. The state of medicine is so bad for physicians that we need a group of thought leaders to build a model that states the first step in prioritizing physician wellness is to make sure that doctors can be human. You know...things like eating, drinking, sleeping, taking care of their family, and having time to urinate. How did we get to the place where we need institutions and think tanks to tell us that taking care of ourselves is important?

---

8    Daniel Shapiro et al., "Beyond Burnout: A Physician Wellness Hierarchy Designed to Prioritize Interventions at the Systems Level," *The American Journal of Medicine* 132, no. 5 (May 2019): 556–63, https://doi.org/10.1016/j. amjmed.2018.11.028.

# Health Professional Wellness Hierarchy

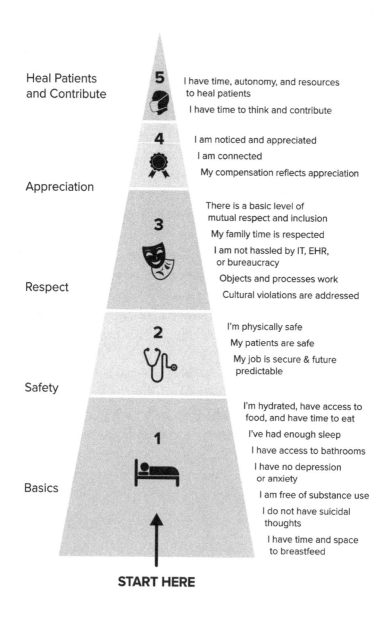

**Heal Patients and Contribute**

**5**

I have time, autonomy, and resources to heal patients

I have time to think and contribute

**4**

I am noticed and appreciated

I am connected

My compensation reflects appreciation

**Appreciation**

**3**

There is a basic level of mutual respect and inclusion

My family time is respected

I am not hassled by IT, EHR, or bureaucracy

Objects and processes work

Cultural violations are addressed

**Respect**

**2**

I'm physically safe

My patients are safe

My job is secure & future predictable

**Safety**

**1**

I'm hydrated, have access to food, and have time to eat

I've had enough sleep

I have access to bathrooms

I have no depression or anxiety

I am free of substance use

I do not have suicidal thoughts

I have time and space to breastfeed

**Basics**

**START HERE**

We arrived here because we work in a system that is broken. Medicine is in major need of change. We must note, however, that this goal of systemic change is not mutually exclusive with the idea of helping physicians defeat burnout and create a life they love. We can, and should, be doing both. While we all recognize the need for the medical system to change, I, for one, refuse to sit idly by, waiting for that system to change while burned-out doctors need help.

As Maya Angelou, the amazing author and native of my hometown in Winston-Salem, put it:

> You should be angry. You must not be bitter. Bitterness is like cancer. It eats upon the host. It doesn't do anything to the object of its displeasure. So use that anger. You write it. You paint it. You dance it. You march it. You vote it. You do everything about it. You talk it. Never stop talking it.[9]

My friends, you should be angry about our broken medical system, but we don't have to let it make us feel bitter, broken, and burned out. On this much, Mandela and Angelou agree. This false dichotomy that many would make between burnout and moral injury is not necessary. Let's fix the morally injurious medical system while we also work toward helping the physicians who are burned out by it.

## THE THREE PILLARS OF BURNOUT

As mentioned above, "burnout" was first described by the German-born psychologist Herbert Freudenberger. In Freudenberger's 1981

---

9    Maya Angelou, "You should be angry...," Twitter, April 15, 2021, 11:30 a.m., https://twitter.com/drmayaangelou/status/1382717886385561603?lang =en.

book called *Burnout: The High Cost of High Achievement,* he points out three key elements.[10] These are emotional exhaustion, depersonalization (originally called cynicism), and a lack of perceived achievement. When experienced, this triad leads to what Freudenberger called "the extinction of motivation or incentive." If emotional exhaustion, depersonalization, and a lack of accomplishment are the symptoms that lead to a loss of intrinsic motivation, what then is the cause? That brings us back to brushing Anna Ruth's teeth.

On the surface—*of burnout, not Anna Ruth's teeth*—the cause seems multifactorial. The Medscape survey on physician burnout, which is filled out by thousands of physicians each year, asks doctors a series of questions to determine the most common components of their burnout. From the 2021 survey, here are the top five reasons that physicians said they were burned out:

- 58% - Too many bureaucratic tasks
- 37% - Spending too many hours at work
- 37% - Lack of respect from administrators/employers, colleagues, and staff
- 32% - Insufficient compensation/reimbursement
- 28% - Lack of control/autonomy

Others making the list but not quite landing in the top five include the electronic medical record system, lack of respect from patients, and government regulations. What is interesting to note from this list is the fifth cause, a "lack of control/autonomy." A lack of autonomy was noted by 28% of physicians, and 100% of toddlers heard 'round the world, as Anna Ruth taught us earlier. For physicians reading this book, we know that autonomy in medicine is specific

---

10   Herbert Freudenberger, *Burnout: The High Cost of Achievement,* (Garden City, NY: Anchor Press, 1980).

to our ability to care for patients without external force or influence. Surely, this is the definition the Medscape survey was using.

However, autonomy can be defined more broadly. And, I would argue that with a broader definition, a lack of autonomy is actually the overarching theme of the emotional exhaustion experienced by burned-out physicians. In other words, a lack of autonomy is the disease, while emotional exhaustion is the symptom of the disease. A broader definition of autonomy makes this clear. Think about it. The other answers on this list include too many hours at work (the number two cause), which reflects doctors' lack of personal autonomy to determine when they get home. In other words, too many hours at the hospital is indicative of a lack of autonomy, or independence, in doctors' personal lives. Too many bureaucratic tasks (the number one cause) implies that doctors lack control over their professional tasks, too.

If autonomy were broadened to include both a professional *and* personal definition of autonomy, it would be the overwhelming cause of emotional exhaustion seen in the Medscape survey. Yet, you work in medicine. So, I don't have to prove that to you, do I? For those still in disbelief that a lack of autonomy is the overarching cause of the emotional exhaustion seen in burned-out physicians, we don't even have to find a different source to make the case. When asked in the same Medscape survey what would improve their burnout, the same burned-out doctors said, in order, the following:

- 45% - Increased compensation to avoid financial stress
- 42% - More manageable work and schedule
- 39% - Greater respect from administrators/employers, colleagues, or staff
- 35% - Increased control/autonomy

Do you notice a theme? All of these potential solutions are a way for physicians to create more personal and professional autonomy.

This is captured in one of Freudenberger's first descriptions of burnout: "a state of mental and physical exhaustion caused by one's professional life." In this definition, Freudenberger makes it clear that burnout is not caused by the individual who is struggling; it is caused by the oppressive and destructive environment in which they work. Burned-out doctors lack a fundamental need that all human beings require, including Anna Ruth—the need for autonomy. We want to do it by "our-own-big-doctor-selves." When doctors are not in control of how we care for patients or when we get home each day, emotional exhaustion is the end result.

How many doctors miss T-ball and soccer games, recitals, weddings, and funerals? How many of us have felt like we couldn't take a vacation or a break because we couldn't afford the life we purchased in order to make us happy? What about all of the time that charting on the EMR steals from physician families? How many times has a burned-out doctor known what to do for a patient but was unable to because of an EMR, insurance company, hospital policy, or administrator?

In an effort to find happiness, many burned-out doctors decide to change jobs or start a side gig to create more financial freedom. This is despite working sixty hours per week at the hospital. Other doctors joined The Great Resignation during the COVID-19 pandemic. Some retired completely from medicine so that they could finally take back control. Still other burned-out doctors thought about getting additional education or training so that they could transition into a different field.

All of these acts are an attempt by doctors to improve their autonomy. It is no wonder that there are physician Facebook groups that have almost 100,000 doctors in them learning about physician side gigs. Simply put, physicians do not feel like the captain of their own ship. The point is that the emotional exhaustion that burned-out physicians experience is caused by a lack of autonomy. However, this is only a third of the story. Remember, burnout also consists of depersonalization and a perceived lack of accomplishment.

The spirit of depersonalization is a loss of compassion. The word compassion stems from the root words *pati* meaning to suffer and *com* which means with. This is why compassion is often defined as meaning "to suffer with." This is an apt description of depersonalization for the medical community. It's the point at which a physician has lost the ability to suffer with their patients and colleagues. In many ways, depersonalization is a lack of belonging to our common humanity. It is what happens when burned-out doctors view their patients and colleagues as "other."

This loss of compassion, according to Freudenberger's definition, is caused by bad cultures and environments. When we work with burned-out physicians in the Alpha Coaching Experience, there is a theme that is loud and clear—burned-out doctors want administrators to listen. Physicians want to be seen, heard, and valued as members of the team. We have a deep need to belong.

This need to feel like we are appreciated, valued, and a respected member of the team is an intrinsic human need. All of us have this desire to belong, even at work. When doctors forget or don't believe they are a valued part of the communities where they work, depersonalization is the result. This is also captured in the Medscape survey responses where physicians said they wanted greater respect from administrators and patients. Almost half of the physicians in the survey agreed.

Belonging consists of more than feeling like a valued team member, however. It also includes our need to feel connected to a deeper purpose or mission that we are working toward. We want to be a part of something bigger than ourselves. This connection to a deeper purpose is the biggest distinction between a vocation (i.e., a calling or mission) and an occupation (i.e., a job). When this greater purpose is missing, doctors begin to treat medicine much more like a job. A loss of compassion for colleagues and patients is the result.

After experiencing burnout, doctors often carry their lunch pail in, do their work, and then take their lunch pail home. Yet, who can blame these lunch pail doctors? They don't feel like they belong to a deeper purpose.

If this wasn't enough, there is a third component to physician burnout—a perceived lack of accomplishment. Isn't it curious, though, that highly accomplished physicians would suffer with this phenomenon? It turns out that up to 60% of physicians suffer from imposter syndrome,[11] or a perceived lack of competence. This is why in 2019, Gottlieb and colleagues looked into potential causes of physician imposter syndrome. What they found was that low self-esteem (i.e., confidence) and bad institutional culture were associated with higher rates of imposter syndrome. Whereas, "social support, validation of success, positive affirmation, and both personal and shared reflections" were shown to be protective against the perceived lack of competence seen in imposter syndrome.

If the conclusion here is that burnout is caused by a lack of autonomy, belonging, and perceived competence, then it turns out the solution to burnout is the opposite: empower physicians to reclaim their autonomy, create communities where doctors feel a deep sense of belonging, and increase perceived competence. Fortunately, there is a name for this group of doctors who have found autonomy, belonging, and competence. They are called self-determined physicians.

---

11   Michael Gottlieb et al., "Impostor Syndrome among Physicians and Physicians in Training: A Scoping Review," *Medical Education* 54, no. 2 (February 2020): 116–24, https://doi.org/10.1111/medu.13956.

# CHAPTER 2

# The ABCs of Self-Determined Physicians

"Control leads to compliance; autonomy leads to engagement."
—Daniel H. Pink

IN THE 1970S, Air New Zealand began offering Antarctic tours to their passengers. They were a big hit. Each passenger paid around $400, or ~$2,000 in today's money, to board this round-trip flight. It was a first-class affair that offered passengers a chance to see things that they had never experienced before. The flight included views of the coast of New Zealand and breathtaking vantage points of the Antarctic as the plane flew over the McMurdo Sound, a large body of water adjacent to the Antarctic. The best part? It all came from the comfort of your own luxury seat without having to brave the Antarctic weather.

It was on November 28, 1979, that Captain Jim Collins left Auckland aboard Air New Zealand Flight 901 for the most famous Air New Zealand Antarctic tour to date. Clouds were covering much of the view that day. So with champagne flutes in their hand, it was about four hours later that the passengers' excitement increased as Captain Jim Collins began his descent so that these well-paying passengers could get the best view. Flight 901 performed two large loops over the McMurdo Sound. As the passengers waited with bated breath, the clouds finally began to break. The excitement at what they were about to see was palpable in the air.

With a plan to descend to two thousand feet to provide the best vantage point, it was at this moment that the ground proximity warning system (GPWS) began to alarm in the cockpit of Flight 901. Captain Jim Collins and copilot Greg Cassi were confused. How in the world could the ground proximity alarm be going off if they were two thousand feet over the McMurdo Sound? Yet, the GPWS alarmed.

The flight recorder caught the moment of the impact. Then, silence.

On that fateful day in 1979 aboard Flight 901, a total of 237 passengers and 20 crew perished. There were only six seconds between the ground proximity warning system alarming and the plane colliding with Mount Erebus, an active volcano that stood at a height of almost 12,500 feet. Only six seconds between excitement and disaster.

Like many, you may be wondering how this happened. What led to the death of 257 people that day when Air New Zealand had been completing these Antarctic trips for over two years without incident? How is it possible that the crew thought that they were heading to a beautiful view over the McMurdo Sound, only to impact an active volcano twenty-seven miles east of their intended destination?

It turned out that the answer was a change in coordinates, placed by the aviation officer at Air New Zealand that morning in an attempt to fix a previous typing error in the system. The change to the coordinates was small. Yet, the consequences were devastating. In aviation, there is a well-described law called the "1 in 60" rule, which states that for every one degree that a plane deviates from its intended coordinate, it will be off by one mile from its target for every sixty miles that it flies. For example, a flight from LAX in Los Angeles to JFK in New York would be off by more than forty miles if the target coordinate was changed by only one degree. That's not a big deal if you are willing to land in the town of Sleepy Hollow or Greenwich, Connecticut, instead of the Big Apple.

Given that the target for Air New Zealand Flight 901 was slightly off the intended path, the flight ended up being twenty-seven miles east of its desired location four hours later. The cloud cover on November 28, 1979, made it impossible to see the volcano that would not have been there if they were where they were supposed to be. Yet, they weren't where they were supposed to be, and their view was a total whiteout. As the plane dropped below the cloud cover so that passengers could have a better view of the landmarks, they were not over the body of water known as the McMurdo Sound as they believed. Instead, they were twenty-seven miles east, where Mount Erebus stands. To this day, the Mount Erebus accident remains New Zealand's worst peacetime tragedy.

There is a lesson to be learned here: deviating even slightly from our intended course can have grave consequences. Even when well-intentioned, being slightly off our intended target in the short term can cost us greatly in the long run. The difference may seem small in the beginning, but it can prove deadly if maintained for a long period of time. Medicine is learning the same lesson after years of administrators' well-meaning yet misplaced focus, and we are now at a watershed moment because of it. The alarms are sounding, and we are now faced with a choice if we want to avoid medicine's Mount Erebus.

## AN EXTINCTION OF MOTIVATION

For years, the focus of most health care organizations has been on maintaining profit. In fact, a common mantra that is often quoted by administrators is, "If there is no margin, then there is no mission!" This is the line of logic that many leaders use to defend a profit-first model. *Who cares how happy our healthcare workers are if we can't turn the lights on? Wouldn't they be less happy if they were unemployed?*

Is it the chicken or the egg? Should the focus be placed on profit in healthcare so that we can, in turn, take care of the people? Or is the opposite true—that when we take care of the healthcare workers on the front line, profit is the inevitable result? It may seem like splitting hairs here, but like Flight 901 taught us, if the destination isn't spot on, the consequence can prove deadly. In this case, a focus on profit over people has led to a complete and profound extinction of motivation in 50% of physicians. We are also now seeing cataclysmic rates of depression and suicide in medicine where, on average, a doctor a day dies by suicide.[12]

Remember, it was Freudenberger, the founder of burnout, that said burnout is "the extinction of motivation or incentive." If the end result of burnout is a loss of motivation, it would be worth our time to determine where our motivation comes from in the first place. To understand motivation, we need to discuss the two different types of motivation that exist: extrinsic and intrinsic motivation.

In medicine, we are provided an incentive if we meet our goals, or a consequence if we don't. The carrots of extrinsic motivation include compensation through increased salaries or from an incentive or bonus structure that rewards us when we achieve metrics provided by our employer or practice. These carrots may also include awards, accolades, or public recognition. In marketing, carrots can be seen in "buy one, get one" (i.e., BOGO) sales or the 10% off MSRP sales that

---

12    Claudia Center et al., "Confronting Depression and Suicide in Physicians: A Consensus Statement," *JAMA* 289, no. 23 (June 2003): 3161–66, https://doi.org/10.1001/jama.289.23.3161.

plaster TV screens for the newest car or truck. In sports and entertainment, the carrot may look like a trophy or a platinum record.

If rewards, bonuses, and public recognition serve as the carrot side of extrinsic motivation, the stick is a negative extrinsic motivator. These sticks include things like quality holdbacks when imposed metrics aren't met. It also includes the money lost when the Centers for Medicare & Medicaid Services, or CMS, queries charts and finds some percentage of our charts not meeting their standards. In some hospital cultures, it may also include public shaming or threats of job loss when certain goals are not met.

Intrinsic motivation, on the other hand, comes from an internal source that compels us to do a good job for the sake of doing a good job. Intrinsic motivation is the form of engagement that hospital administrators want but seem to have a never-ending penchant to diminish. Daniel H. Pink, the author of the book *Drive: The Surprising Truth About What Motivates Us,* says the following about intrinsic motivation: "Human beings have an innate inner drive to be autonomous, self-determined, and connected to one another. And when that drive is liberated, people achieve more and live richer lives."

When Freudenberger referred to burnout causing a lack of motivation, he was likely referring to the extinction of intrinsic motivation described here by Daniel Pink. Pink's vantage point in *Drive* is rooted in the research performed in the 1970s by Edward Deci (pronounced "DC") and Richard Ryan, who first described what is known today as Self-Determination Theory.[13] Self-Determination Theory consists of three key elements—autonomy, relatedness (which I'll call "belonging"), and competence. You can think of these as the ABCs of Self-Determination Theory. Let's look at each of these in turn.

---

13   To learn more about SDT, I'd highly encourage you to read *Drive* by Daniel H. Pink or to visit https://selfdeterminationtheory.org/.

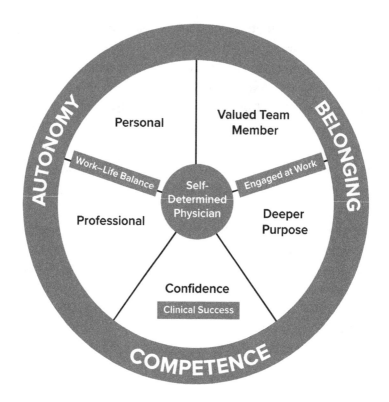

## AUTONOMY

Personal autonomy is the freedom to choose how we live our life without undue influence or coercion. This definition of autonomy implies that we have control over our schedule and our destiny in life. If we want to make the T-ball game or the recital, we are able to do that. When there is a date with our spouse on the calendar, we aren't running late for the forty-seventh time because we were stuck at the hospital or clinic again.

However, autonomy extends to patient care, too. Professional autonomy, then, is the ability to take care of our patients however we feel it is best without the impediment of administrators, insurance companies, or systems preventing us from providing that care.

The only influence that takes place is that of the patient, who also has autonomy that must be protected.

When filtered through this lens, it is easy to see why many burned-out physicians experience the extinction of intrinsic motivation. From our inability to know exactly when we will get home, to the boxes that must be checked in order to make sure we get reimbursed for our care, very little is left up to the physician on the front line in terms of how to perform our job. Then there are the preauthorizations and approvals doctors must complete for insurance companies, pharmaceutical staff, or administrators prior to providing the diagnosis and treatment modalities that patients need. This doesn't even include the bevy of systematic limitations caused by the electronic medical record systems.

Interestingly, studies show that there is a link between extrinsic (carrot-and-stick) motivators and autonomy. It turns out that when people receive external rewards and punishment, we feel pushed or pulled by the reward rather than by an innate drive to do what is right. Said differently, extrinsic motivators diminish our autonomy. This holds true with financial rewards, too. In fact, once we are earning a fair wage, monetary rewards fail to improve our engagement and intrinsic motivation. Behavioral economics studies indicate that increased salaries do not increase our long-term satisfaction or sense of well-being, either. After being paid a fair wage, any additional carrot-or-stick motivation through monetary means actually diminishes our levels of engagement. The reason is that the metrics to receive the reward are imposed by authority figures outside of us rather than by intrinsic and autonomous goals from inside.

Like Anna Ruth, we all want to do it by our own big-girl (and big-boy) selves. This innate need for autonomy has been studied in a vast array of disciplines. Two large-scale studies with over 6,000 and 8,000 people published in the *Vaccine* journal showed that a lack of autonomy has been linked to lower rates of vaccination to

COVID-19 when individuals are mandated to get a vaccine.[14] While I'm not saying that I am against vaccine mandates, I am saying that mandating that someone else do something is an attack on their autonomy. And we should not be surprised when people balk. At our core, human beings do not like being told what to do.

A lack of autonomy and physician well-being has also been established in medicine. In a study published in *Medical Care Research and Review* assessing over 2,000 physicians utilizing the AMA Physician Masterfile,[15] researchers from the University of Illinois found that decreasing autonomy was associated with increased rates of burnout, depression, and an intention to leave medical practice. However, when autonomy improved, it was associated with increased rates of well-being at work. Intrinsic motivation was shown to be protective against deteriorating occupational health. The more autonomy physicians have, the more likely we are to have better health.

## BELONGING (A.K.A. RELATEDNESS)

In the now-infamous Milgram experiment, Stanley Milgram—a Yale psychologist—studied the connection between obedience and psychology. With World War II freshly in mind, Milgram's 1963 study looked into how otherwise normal German citizens could become complicit in genocide of the Jewish people. In other words, why would otherwise good people do such terrible things?

---

14   Mathias Schmitz et al., "Predicting vaccine uptake during COVID-19 crisis: A motivational approach," *Vaccine* 40, no. 2 (January 2021): 288–97, https://doi.org/10.1016/j.vaccine.2021.11.068.

15   Arlen Moller et al., "Motivational Mechanisms Underlying Physicians' Occupational Health: A Self-Determination Theory Perspective," *Medical Care Research and Review* 79, no. 2 (April 2021): 255–66, https://doi.org/10.1177/10775587211007748.

In Milgram's study, participants were invited to draw names from a hat to determine whether they would play the role of "learner" or "teacher." Unbeknownst to them, the odds were fixed. The learner role was always played by a preselected member or actor of the research team. The research participants were always slated to be the "teacher" in the Milgram experiment. For their participation, they were promised to be paid $4.50, which is equivalent to about $20 today.

The teacher, in a separate room from the learner, was then instructed to utilize a switchboard that consisted of a row of switches that provided an electrical shock via leads attached to the learner. The switches were all labeled. The first switch was fifteen volts and was labeled "Slight Shock." The switches continued into the middle of the switchboard to 375 volts, which was labeled "Severe Shock." Finally, on the other end was a 450-volt switch which was labeled "XXX." This indicated it was a lethal voltage.

The experiment also involved a third person, dressed in a white coat, who facilitated the test. In Milgram's study, the learners were asked to recall certain words. When they made a mistake, the participants were instructed to apply a shock to the learner. With each incorrect answer, the research participants would administer an increasingly severe shock. If the participant expressed a desire to stop shocking the learner, the authoritarian figure in the white coat prodded them with certain predetermined responses. The first time participants asked to stop the experiment, they would be instructed to "Please continue." With the second, third, and fourth attempts, they were respectively told, "The experiment requires that you continue"; "It is absolutely essential that you continue"; and "You have no other choice, you must go on."

The research participant was instructed at the beginning that they could stop at any point. They were also told that the researcher in the white lab coat could not press the switch for them. Yet, 65% of participants walked into the experiment thinking they were a good person, only to find out that for just $20, they were willing to administer a lethal shock of 450 volts to someone else if an authority figure told them they must continue. Pretty alarming, isn't it?

In a variation of the Milgram experiment that is more germane to our discussion, participants were placed in a variety of locations while performing the same experiment. While the first part of the experiment focused on the impact of an authoritarian figure, this variation of the experiment focused on the proximity to the individual being shocked. In other words, would physical distance impact someone's willingness to administer a lethal shock?

In the original experiment the teacher was in a separate room from the learner. In that setting, 65% of participants administered a lethal shock. In this new experiment, participants were first seated in the same room as the learner. They could see and hear people scream as they received the shocks. When in closer proximity to the learner, the percentage of participants willing to administer a lethal shock dropped from 65% to 40%. In the most extreme example of proximity, participants were required to physically place the other person's hand on a shock plate. Then, they remained in the same room while administering the exam. This more intimate setting led to even lower rates of completion, where participants' willingness to administer a lethal shock was cut in half from 65% to 30%.

While Milgram's experiment is considered highly controversial and unethical since it taught people they'd be willing to murder someone else in the right conditions for just twenty bucks, there are a couple of clear takeaways from this work. The first is that even good people, when placed into a bad culture, will do bad things, including administering a lethal shock to someone else. This is called ethical fading, where people will behave contrary to their perceived set of morals while maintaining that they are good people. This is what happens in bad cultures. Particularly when instructed to do so by an authoritarian figure. When someone lets authoritarian figures steal their agency, they become agents of the system instead of autonomous beings and, therefore, have the potential to be complicit in genocide like German citizens were during World War II.

The second point we can learn from Milgram's experiment is that the further distanced we are from the people we work with, the more likely it is that we would be willing to cause harm to them. Said differently, the closer we are to someone physically and emotionally, the less likely we are to cause them harm. This explains how healthcare administrators, who are otherwise well-meaning people, can cause great harm to the medical professionals they lead. As healthcare leaders lack proximity to burned-out medical professionals on the front line, any connection they may have once felt can be lost.

There is precedent here as well. In 2015, Valeant Pharmaceuticals (now known as Bausch Health) found itself in hot water after price-gouging patients. Valeant was caught raising prices on drugs, including the diabetes medication Glumetza. Valeant also misled investors after setting up a mail-order pharmacy and price-hiking drugs after acquiring smaller pharmaceutical companies. For example, when Valeant purchased Marathon Pharmaceuticals, the manufacturer of cardiac medications like Isuprel and Nitropress, it subsequently increased the prices of these two drugs by 500% and 200%, respectively. What likely started out as a company meant to help patients with their medical problems turned into a company where the CEO, Michael Pearson, was so far removed from the patients he was trying to help, ethical fading became prominent. This eventually led to the heinous act of making necessary medications unaffordable for many patients.

After being sanctioned by the Securities and Exchange Commission (SEC) and appearing before the US Congress, Pearson apologized for inappropriately raising the prices of drugs and for failing to disclose their connection to the mail-order pharmacy they created. In the end, this cost Valeant $45 million. A slap on the wrist for a company of Valeant's size. Pearson was required to pay $250,000 in penalties to the SEC and $450,000 to Valeant.

Milgram's experiment continues to ring true more than sixty years later as CEOs and leaders in healthcare are distanced from their healthcare professionals and the patients they serve.

The bad cultures and lack of proximity serve as an affront to the second element of Self-Determination Theory: "belonging." Belonging, which is called relatedness in psychological literature, describes our natural human tendency toward integrated work with others who share a common vision. This has two parts: being part of a team and sharing a deeper vision.

The first portion of belonging means that we feel like we have caring relationships where people value and appreciate us. In other words, belonging happens when we have the sort of environment and culture where we feel safe to share our worries and concerns. This is an environment where our voices are heard. We feel like valued members of the team and feel that we are contributing in a meaningful way. We are safe and in close proximity to those that lead us.

Unsurprisingly, this need to be a part of a team has been borne out in sports literature, where belonging has been shown to be dependent not only on a teammate's relationships with their peers, but also with the leader of the team, the coach.[16] In the previously mentioned study on physician autonomy from the University of Illinois, Moller and colleagues argue that doctors need to be on the same team as their patients and the healthcare system. They argue further that the loss of insurance for patients in the United States undermines physician well-being because physicians sometimes feel like they are not on the same team as their patients. The physician wants to provide the best care while uninsured patients are

---

16    Tsz Lun Chu and Tao Zhang, "The Roles of Coaches, Peers, and Parents in Athletes' Basic Psychological Needs: A Mixed-Studies Review," *International Journal of Sports Science and Coaching* 14, no. 4 (July 2019), https://doi. org/10.1177/1747954119858458.

often more concerned with the cost. Values are not aligned because of a bad insurance environment. As we have learned, good people can do bad things in such an environment. This lack of belonging has a deep impact on the depersonalization seen in burned-out physicians.

There is a second piece to our definition of belonging. Belonging also includes our need to be connected to a deeper sense of purpose in our world. In other words, belonging can be described as our need to have impact. It is important for people to feel that the team's mission is more important than any single individual, including themselves. The most successful military units get this. From the Navy Seals to the Army Rangers, these specialized units all have a deep sense of belonging to their brothers and sisters in arms. They eat together, live together, and fight together, all while trying to accomplish a goal that is much bigger than any one of them alone. In other words, they are not only in close proximity with each other, but also with their purpose.

This begs the question then, what is the deeper purpose of the office, clinic, or hospital where you work? What is the overarching goal that the team seems to be working toward? Have your department chair, CEO, or other leaders ever expressly stated a vision and how we might go about getting there? Have we been granted the autonomy to achieve that goal with our well-earned abilities, energy, and talent? Or are we simply instructed that "we must continue" even when we want to stop?

The answer is that these leaders likely haven't provided this vision at all. And, even when they do, the words they utter stand in stark contrast to the actions we see as physicians on the front line. This is why doctors don't feel a deep-seated connection to our administrators and leaders. It is more than a lack of shared vision, though. A disconnection from the leaders that lead us proves costly, too. Just like in Milgram's experiment, where physical distance led to great harm.

It is no wonder then why physicians feel like they do not belong on a team where, if we are being honest, the CEO, CMO, COO, and C-Whatever-Else-O wouldn't even recognize us if they passed us on the street. Proximity is nonexistent. Unlike the Navy Seals or Army Rangers, most of our leaders haven't been in the trenches with the doctors they are meant to protect. Even when they do occasionally visit, administrators have a curated experience when they enter into our world. This separation from our leaders both physically and emotionally causes great discord. It also leads to an easy target for the working physician to blame for all of their woes. Even more worrisome, as seen in the Milgram experiment, this distance between physicians and their leaders makes it possible for administrators who are otherwise good people to administer a lethal culture that saps physicians of their sense of autonomy and belonging, which is far too often experienced today.

As Simon Sinek, a thought leader and author of the must-read book entitled *Leaders Eat Last,* points out:

> If our leaders are to enjoy the trappings of their position in the hierarchy, then we expect them to offer us protection. The problem is, for many of the overpaid leaders, we know that they [take] the money and perks and [don't] offer protection to their people. In some cases, they even sacrificed their people to protect or boost their own interests. This is what so viscerally offends us. We [the employees] only accuse them of greed and excess when we feel they have violated the very definition of what it means to be a leader.

It is this lack of belonging and protection that Sinek points to that leads many physicians to experience the lack of belonging that is so prevalent in burned-out physicians. Doctors feel more like the learner getting shocked in the Milgram experiment than like a valued and respected team member. And we certainly do not share a common vision with those that are paid to lead the way.

## PERCEIVED COMPETENCE

We have discussed the autonomy and belonging of Self-Determination. However, there is a third component of Self-Determination Theory called "competence." Competence can be described as the measure of our mastery or skill in our profession. When we feel this perceived mastery (i.e., clinical confidence), it can serve as a powerful driver for intrinsic motivation.

Competence, then, in medicine occurs when a physician feels that they have mastered both the art and science of caring for patients. While none of us may truly reach mastery given the continually changing landscape of healthcare (*we call it "practicing" medicine for a reason*), feeling confident and competent are an important component of becoming a self-determined physician.

Self-determination is making its way into the medical literature as well, where educators have been tasked with creating ways to foster autonomy, belonging, and competence in their physicians-in-training. In an article from James Wagner published in *Medical Teacher*, Wagner and his colleagues demonstrated that there are two crucial factors that lead to job satisfaction in medical school learning communities.[17] The first is campus engagement, which can be described as an improved sense of community. This ties back into our previous discussion on belonging. The second component Wagner calls for includes skill development, which allows learners to feel like a better doctor. In other words, when we feel like we are competent

---

17    James Michael Wagner et al., "Benefits to Faculty Involved in Medical School Learning Communities," *Medical Teacher* 37, no. 5 (May 2015): 476–81, https://doi.org/10.3109/0142159X.2014.947940.

at what we do, it produces engagement. And being engaged allows us to continually work toward becoming a better doctor in active teaching environments seen in medical schools.

We also see the opposite of perceived competence in healthcare, which is called imposter syndrome, a lack of confidence or the belief that you aren't as good as others, despite outward objective evidence that argues to the contrary. For doctors, particularly those young in their career or those who are stepping into a new leadership role, imposter syndrome is a very real phenomenon that saps their ability to enjoy their work. When a bad patient outcome occurs, they are likely to blame it on themselves, even if the outcome had little to do with their decisions or care. As the comedian Demetri Martin points out, "Saying 'I'm sorry' and 'I apologize' are the same thing. Except at a Funeral." Unfortunately, to doctors suffering from imposter syndrome, this might not seem funny at all. In order to be self-determined, physicians must be confident in their clinical abilities. In this way, there is a marriage between confidence and competence that produces the third and final element of self-determination.

## BURNOUT AND SELF-DETERMINATION

We have established that burned-out physicians experience emotional exhaustion which stems from a lack of personal and professional autonomy. Self-determined physicians, on the other hand, are completely autonomous in both settings. Burned-out physicians suffer from depersonalization, which is caused by a loss of belonging and compassion. Self-determined physicians have a deep and meaningful sense of belonging to both their team and the deeper purpose within these communities. Finally, burned-out physicians lack a sense of accomplishment or ability, while the self-determined physician has complete confidence and is competent in their work.

You can see that the burned-out physician and the self-determined physician are on polar ends of a spectrum. If burnout is the disease, then the healthiest state is being self-determined. Our goal then is to create systems and cultures that foster self-determined physicians who can experience autonomy, belonging, and competence in medicine. I would contend that this work needs to occur at both the institutional and individual level. Only then can we tear down the systemic and systematic causes in medicine that lead to physician burnout. In order to do this, medicine must shift its focus away from a profit-over-people model and create cultures and environments that value people over profit.

# CHAPTER 3

# People over Profit

"When something is important enough, you do it
even if the odds are not in your favor."
—Elon Musk

JAMES BLAKE WAS born on April 14, 1912. He was drafted into the Army in 1943. After his service, Blake found employment as a bus driver in Montgomery, Alabama, during the 1950s, when bus drivers did more than transport passengers from one destination to another. Montgomery bus drivers in the 1950s were also granted police powers to enforce local laws and policies.

While driving his bus, Blake first made waves when he ran Lucille Times—a Black woman—off the road multiple times while she was on the way to the dry cleaners. After entering into a bit of road rage, Blake eventually cut off Lucille Times's car such that she could not move forward. Blake then exited the bus and began berating Ms. Times, calling her a "black son of a bitch." After she told Blake that made him a "white son of a bitch," a fight developed between James Blake and Lucille Times. This continued until two motorcycle-riding police officers broke up the fight, and one of the officers told

Times, "If you were a man, I'd beat your head to jelly" for starting a fight with a white man.[18]

Blake's altercation with Times was one of the inciting events that would lead to his more famous encounter with Rosa Parks.[19] It was on December 1, 1955, when Rosa Parks boarded Blake's Montgomery bus after a long day at work and claimed her seat in the "colored" section. The bus was crowded that day, and so it was at another stop that a white man entered the bus, only to find that the "white" section was full. That's when Blake decided that at least one of the rows in the "colored" section would need to be cleared for white passengers.

Blake then demanded that the four Black passengers sitting in the first row of the colored section should stand up and move to the back of the bus. The Black passengers in Montgomery had experienced the segregation laws on these buses many times. This was not a new circumstance. More than one Black rider that day decided it wasn't worth it to fight the fight. They got up and moved to the back.

However, Rosa Parks was sitting in this section too, and she wasn't going to move. Parks had had enough. While the other three Black passengers complied with Blake's demands, Rosa Parks did not. As the secretary for the National Association for the Advancement of Colored People, or NAACP, she was well aware of the incidents occurring on the Montgomery bus line at the time, including Blake's previous altercation with Lucille Times. And she was tired of it all. Rosa decided that she was done with the victim mindset that so many friends and family carried with them during those times.

---

18 "Lucille Times obituary," *The New York Times*, August 22, 2021, https://www.nytimes.com/2021/08/22/obituaries/lucille-times-dead.html.
19 "Rosa Parks," History.com, January 19, 2022, https://www.history.com/topics/black-history/rosa-parks.

Instead, Parks found the courage and power to stand up for what she knew was right. She could tolerate the consequences. What she could not tolerate anymore was continuing to exist in a racist environment. The Jim Crow segregation era had done nothing for her and her friends except cause pain.

On that day in 1955, Rosa Parks demonstrated that it is possible to refuse to be the victim of an external circumstance while simultaneously serving as the hero of our story. Rosa Parks refused to feel helpless. She stood up for the change she knew needed to happen. She reclaimed her autonomy despite the odds being heavily stacked against her. Did Rosa Parks have some superpower that day that allowed her to stay cool, calm, and collected in a situation that saw most people crumble under the pressure? No, but she did understand what many others have taught us—that we can fight for our autonomy while we refuse to let external situations cause us internal harm.

What then can burned-out doctors learn from Rosa Parks's example? We can learn that just because the healthcare system continually puts medical professionals last, that doesn't mean we have to let it happen. When we get moved to the back of the bus because we are told that other things are more important, we do not have to listen. We can stay cool, calm, and collected while we wage war against online modules, preauthorizations for insurance, EMR charting requirements, administrators, and insurance companies. Just like Rosa.

Most caring physicians believe that "the patient comes first," yet I think this is one of the most outdated beliefs in medicine. If you put everything and everyone else first in medicine, does that really result in the great patient care that everyone wants? No, it doesn't. In fact, when doctors continually let the system beat them down and move them to the back of the medical system's bus in order to put everyone else first, it causes great harm.

It is like the airline industry teaches us every time we board a flight. They tell us to put on our own oxygen mask *first* before helping others to do the same. Why? Because, if we don't put our mask on and we pass out from hypoxia, then we won't be able to help anyone. It is exactly the same in medicine—we cannot pour from an empty cup. As hardworking and caring doctors, we must take care of ourselves first in order to provide the best care to our patients. This is exactly what the People First framework we will discuss below teaches us. Individual physicians can claim this People First focus, whether their healthcare organizations have done the same or not.

It is important work to learn how to refuse to be the victim of a broken system. However, it is equally important to learn Rosa Parks's lesson that we can harness that same power and still stand up for the change we know is right. The change doctors need. And remember, we aren't just standing up for ourselves. We are standing up for our patients, too.

In order to do this, we must learn how to stand up and fight the broken system. Like Parks, we can do the internal thought work necessary to live a life above reproach despite terrible circumstances and also realize when it is time to fight back against external circumstances. She did this from a place of strength, not scarcity. Doctors need to do the same.

## WATERSHED MOMENT

In the United States, there is a nursing shortage that is expected to continue into 2030.[20] These estimated shortages were only exacerbated by the COVID-19 pandemic. With an increasing number of ailing patients, and a dramatically declining nursing force, this caused major issues for hospital systems. Profit-focused hospitals with

---

20  Edward Mehdaova, "Strategies to Overcome the Nursing Shortage," (doctoral dissertation, Walden University, 2017), https://scholarworks.waldenu.edu/cgi/viewcontent.cgi?article=5933&context=dissertations.

a keen eye on their balance sheets quickly filled up any employed nursing shortages they had by paying travel nurses. According to an article on the website Advisory Board, some staffing agencies saw a 284% increase in travel nursing demands two years after the beginning of the pandemic.[21]

Due to the economic pressures caused by supply and demand during the pandemic, some traveling nurses made high four- and sometimes five-figure wages per week. For example, in December 2021, Vivian, a company responsible for finding nursing jobs, offered a position making $9,125 per week for sixty hours of work. At this rate, for only twenty-six weeks of work per year, a travel nurse pursuing opportunities like this could make well over $200,000 annually.

While working sixty hours per week is well above the norm for nursing, sixty hours per week is right around the average number of hours most physicians work. Yet, a salary of more than $200,000 annually is on par with—and even dwarfs—some physician specialties. These $200,000 annual salaries also outcompete many with more advanced nursing-based degrees, including nurse practitioners and CRNAs. The worst part of it all, however, is that these higher payments led to a bidding war and eventually began to tear apart hospital cultures. When independently contracted travel nurses are paid much higher wages than the employed nurses who are already working at the hospital, bitterness is the natural consequence. In other words, it is not sustainable for the employed "local" nurses to perform the same exact job with the same exact credentials in a room adjacent to these highly paid travel nurses, while making a fraction of the pay. It is a direct affront on their need

21  "Helpful or Hurtful? The 'Double-Edged Sword' of Travel Nursing," Advisory Board, September 20, 2021, https://www.advisory.com/daily-briefing/2021/09/20/travel-nurses.

to feel valued and appreciated. Eventually, these local nurses will no longer feel that deep sense of belonging that we all require.

While hiring traveling nurses does, in fact, fill a short-term need for many hospitals, it comes at a very high long-term cost. When employed nurses were paid less by their home institution for the same work, many decided to make a change. Some changed jobs to get paid more. Other employed nurses wised up to this imbalance and became travel nurses themselves, only to come back to the same hospital where they were previously employed. Then, they performed the same exact job in the exact same location for the same employer and were paid three to four times what they were previously making.

In reality, hospitals were often paying substantially more for the same nursing care from the same human being. This may have gone unnoticed in hospitals where employees are a number on a balance sheet. While traveling nurses may have alleviated staffing shortages in the short term, paying substantially more for these temporary medical professionals also had the potential to destroy long-term cultures. Administrators often justified the decision to hire travel nurses or other short-term staff by pointing out that they had no choice. Unless they wanted to keep hemorrhaging money from lost patient care, they had to pay for travel nurses in order to staff the floor and ICU beds. Yet, is this really what happens in the long run? Do the hospitals who hire temporary staff stop hemorrhaging money and make profit in the long run?

Of course, the answer is often no. Many hospitals that put Band-Aids on the nursing shortage in order to salvage profit ended up in a bidding war. Paying physician salaries to nurses is unsustainable. This all has the downstream impact of destroying the value of advanced-practice providers and physicians, and it is all a result of focusing on short-term profit over long-term cultures.

The lesson here is that while a focus on profit may fix numbers in the short term, it often has devastating consequences in the long term. Like Air New Zealand Flight 901 that may not have started very far from its intended flight path, with passing time, it veered more and more off course until it collided with a volcano. By placing its focus on short-term profits instead of long-term cultures, medicine is heading toward its own disaster. Instead of playing the long game that is focused on the autonomy, belonging, and competence of their employees, organizations that focus on the quarterly or annual balance sheets will eventually fold.

The nursing shortage ended up being a direct attack on the ABCs of Self-Determination (representing Autonomy, Belonging, and Competence). It turns out that it gets old having to hire the third nanny after a CRNA has to pick up another unexpected shift or is forced to stay later than usual. Again. This prevents them from having personal autonomy in their life. When hospitals stop caring about autonomy, healthcare professionals leave. When we view these medical professionals like cogs in the wheel, we are waging war against any value they require as a member of the team, too. When people are just numbers on a balance sheet, the answer may seem easy in the short term. We can always find more nurses, they say! At least cases are getting done in the operating rooms, right? Right. Until they aren't, because they all left after we destroyed their autonomy and sense of belonging.

While the nursing shortage example focuses specifically on nurses, the same line of logic applies to any medical professionals, including advanced-practice providers and physicians. Like in Milgram's experiment, administrators in profit-margin-focused hospitals are *not* bad people. The problem happens when our leaders have very little proximity to the healthcare professionals on the front line. A focus on the monthly profit and loss sheet may allow organizations to make the quarterly budget. Annual financial goals might even be met. However, the collateral damage from this framework is seen downstream, when the ripple effect of burned-out medical professionals takes place. When doctors, nurses, and advanced-

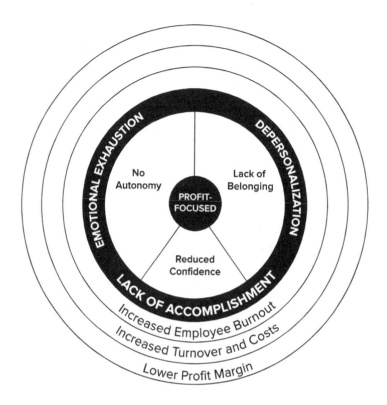

practice providers start leaving their jobs, go part-time, or quit medicine altogether, who will care for patients then? How much profit will it create when we cannot care for the increasing volume of patients? When we have to shut down operating rooms because we cannot find the people to staff them? This race to zero is a losing game for everyone. And it only worsens the existing physician and nursing shortage, ultimately driving up the costs and lowering the profits of the institution.

## THE HEALTHCARE CULTURE CONTINUUM

Where we put our focus matters. Air New Zealand Flight 901 taught us that. Healthcare leaders can choose to focus on profit. Or people.

Like a randomized controlled trial, leaders only get one primary outcome, unless you want to pay the price of a Bonferroni correction. *Even statistics realizes that two primary outcomes come at a cost.* Other outcomes may be important, but they are secondary. Unfortunately, most organizations choose profit as their primary outcome. As Simon Sinek points out in his book *The Infinite Game*, the primacy placed on profit is not new. In a landmark paper from the 1970s written by Milton Friedman, Sinek explores Friedman's focus on profit over people that remains prevalent today:

> Indeed Friedman insisted that there is one and only one social responsibility of business. To use its resources and engage in activities designed to increase its profits so long as it stays within the rules of the game. In other words, according to Friedman the sole purpose of business is to make money and that money belongs to the shareholders.

By placing the primary emphasis on growing profits instead of focusing on the employees and the culture where employees work, this ironically leads to a lower profit margin in the long run. It is like starting a marathon and running as fast as we possibly can for the first mile. While we may be in first place after that initial mile is complete, we will inevitably end up far behind the others and may not even finish the race. In running, this is called a "fly and die." And this is exactly what happens so often to healthcare organizations that place an emphasis on profit over the consistent and long-term employee-based focus that is required to create solid workplace cultures. They fly and then they die in a merger and acquisition deal, burning out everyone else in the process.

The reason for focusing on profit is more obvious than you might think. Healthcare leaders are no different than any other business leader. Administrators love what they can measure. You know, profit and loss statements, balance sheets, metrics, and surveys.

Leaders choose measurable profits over their people instead of their people over profit because it is more concrete and objective. More importantly, they work in systems that require them to meet their projected budgets and profit margins—or face the possibility of losing their jobs. This misplaced focus is not because administrators are bad people.

Whether they realize it or not, each healthcare organization has a choice. With each decision our leaders make, they are either focusing on people or they are focusing on profit. With each vote that they make in one decision or the other, they are pushing their organization along what I call the Healthcare Culture Continuum. With each vote toward profit, healthcare leaders push their culture to the left on the Healthcare Culture Continuum and toward creating more burned-out physicians. With each vote that places an emphasis on the autonomy, belonging, and competence of their employees, healthcare leaders shift their Healthcare Culture Continuum to the right and toward self-determined physicians. While no organization will get every decision correct, as the votes build up in one direction or the other, a culture will be created. It will either be one that extinguishes the intrinsic motivation of its physicians through burnout, or, more ideally, it will be a culture where physicians experience work-life balance, engagement at work, and the intrinsic motivation to do a good job for a good job's sake.

## SHIFTING THE CULTURE

In an effort to make the abstract more concrete, you may be asking how we can shift our cultures toward the left or toward the right on the Healthcare Culture Continuum. You already have the answer: we can focus on profit, or we can focus on people. To illustrate the downstream impact of these choices, you can find a visual representation of what this might look like below. On the left, you'll see the Profit over People framework employed in most hospitals and organizations that pushes the Healthcare Culture Continuum toward burnout. This is the model hospitals used when they played the short game by paying for travel nurses without worrying about the long-term consequences. It is the one that says, "If we cannot keep the lights on, we cannot pay our employees." As each vote is cast toward the profit model, a culture is created that will inevitably diminish autonomy, belonging, and competence. The end result of this deadly triad is burned-out physicians and nurses. Burnout, in turn, leads to lower engagement and increased physician turnover and cost for healthcare organizations. By shifting the culture toward burnout, this model eventually destroys the very thing it set out to build in the first place—profit.

On the right, you'll see the People First framework, which is the model that—if followed—will shift the Healthcare Culture Continuum to the right. It is the key to changing the culture of medicine and empowering individual physicians, too. With an employee-focused framework, leaders are encouraged to focus on the three basic tenets of self-determination. In turn, this leads to improved cultures and patient outcomes, less physician turnover/cost, and ultimately an increase in the profit margins that healthcare leaders so desperately want. Higher profits are a natural by-product of putting people first.

Oxford defines "focus" as the center of interest or activity. Each hospital has a single and universal focus. Some organizations focus on profit. Others focus on people. However, they cannot focus on both. As the Russian proverb teaches, "If you chase two rabbits, you will not catch either one." The goal of any healthcare organization should be to shift the culture of their workplace toward the right on the continuum, or toward creating self-determined employees. In order to do this, organizations must be laser-focused on creating trusting cultures for their employees. You'll note that saying these are your values and practicing them are not one and the same.

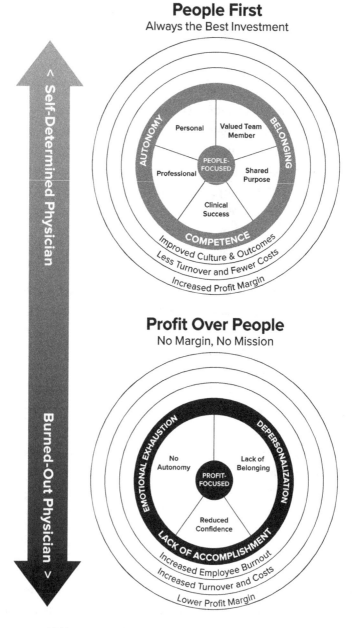

## People First
### Always the Best Investment

**Self-Determined Physician**

PEOPLE-FOCUSED

AUTONOMY
- Personal
- Professional

BELONGING
- Valued Team Member
- Shared Purpose

COMPETENCE
- Clinical Success

Improved Culture & Outcomes
Less Turnover and Fewer Costs
Increased Profit Margin

## Profit Over People
### No Margin, No Mission

**Burned-Out Physician**

PROFIT-FOCUSED

EMOTIONAL EXHAUSTION
- No Autonomy

DEPERSONALIZATION
- Lack of Belonging

LACK OF ACCOMPLISHMENT
- Reduced Confidence

Increased Employee Burnout
Increased Turnover and Costs
Lower Profit Margin

How are healthcare organizations going to hit a target if they do not know where they are aiming? Like asking a large crowd of healthcare administrators at an indoor conference to close their eyes and point north, we should not be surprised when they open their eyes and see others in the auditorium pointing in very different directions. We cannot consistently hit our target of shifting our cultures to the right by mistake. It takes intentional focus. And when leaders intentionally set their sights on serving the healthcare workers that work for them, they feel a bit like P.T. Barnum, shooting for the sun, yet landing amongst the stars.

The People First framework can be applied at both an institutional and individual level. At an institutional level, this employee-focused mindset intends to build cultures and systems that foster autonomy, belonging, and competence. This focus on physician well-being creates a ripple effect shown by the concentric circles outlining the main portion of the framework. When more physicians experience autonomy, belonging, and competence, this will result in more self-determined physicians. Self-determined physicians experience better well-being and higher engagement. This leads to improved cultures and outcomes. In turn, the organization will experience lower turnover and lower costs by reducing the need to hire new faculty or pay for locums or traveling medical professionals, for example. The end result? A higher profit margin. Let's examine the ideal framework more closely.

When the focus is placed on the medical professionals in the trenches, our medical professionals will, in turn, take the best

The Healthcare Culture Continuum shown above is physician-centric. However, this continuum can apply to any medical professional, including advanced-practice providers, nurses, staff, and physicians. The word "provider"—which is universally loathed by all physicians outside of those in leadership—could also be placed at either end of the continuum to describe burned-out "providers" and self-determined "providers," respectively.

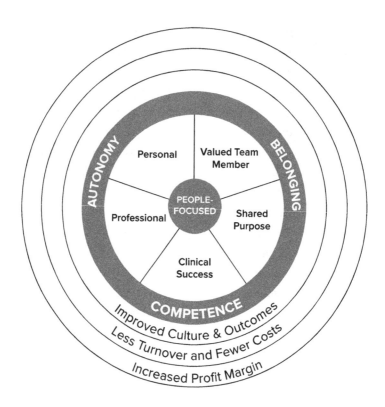

care of the patients and be the best stewards of the organization's resources. This will naturally raise profits as more customer referrals occur while simultaneously driving down cost. This increased profit then leads to a happier board of directors, and the C-suite gets what they want, too. Everyone is happy.

This can all be accomplished when leaders in medicine (and individual physicians) focus on the five components of the People over Profit model. The first two components fall under the "A" of the ABCs of self-determination, or autonomy, and are broken down into personal autonomy and professional autonomy. Any decision that increases these two domains will lead to better work-life balance and a more self-determined physician workforce. The third and fourth components are all about creating environments where people feel like they belong, or the "B" of self-determination. That third component of the employee-focused model is creating an environment where team members feel valued. And the fourth component is allowing those on the team to share a deeper purpose. When healthcare professionals feel like they belong, that is when the engagement happens. Finally, the fifth component is creating cultures where doctors have the confidence that leads to clinical success and competence, the "C" of self-determination. Competence is what produces clinical satisfaction at work.

The five components of the People over Profit framework play the long game. Leaders who focus on increasing these five components understand that when our frontline medical workers are happy, everything else will work out, too. This has been exemplified in other companies outside of medicine that have seen enormous success. Take, for example, a company like Costco. At Costco, they have realized that if they focus on their employees first, the customers will be happy, profits will grow, and then the board of directors and C-suite officers will naturally follow suit. This "employee first" focus explains why Costco boasts a 94% retention rate after one year of employment. Their closest competitor, Sam's Club, which has an infinitely more profit-focused model, has a retention rate of only 56%.

What does this People over Profit focus lead to in concrete terms for employees at Costco? Well, employees receive, on average, a higher base pay than their competitors. Hourly employees have received at least fifteen dollars per hour since 2019 at Costco, well before anyone else raised the minimum wage to that level. And over half of their employees make more than twenty-five dollars per hour. As we discussed previously, extrinsic motivators like increased pay only provide so much benefit. Fortunately for the employees who work at Costco, it is about much more than the pay.

Costco is also closed on Thanksgiving and many other holidays so that employees can spend time with their families. Oh, and their benefits package includes vision and dental coverage in addition to solid healthcare insurance and a good 401(k) program. This explains why one employee told *Business Insider* in an article, "I legitimately love my job." Another added, "Costco is an ideal kind of job."[22]

If Costco were to look at these decisions from a profit-focused model, each of these decisions surely would cost more money in the short term. However, in the big picture, the end result is a better culture and less cost from turnover. Like with physicians, losing an employee and hiring a new one is costly. With a 94% retention rate, Costco rarely has to deal with the high cost of turnover. Because Costco has consistently placed their people over potential profit, they have reaped the rewards of a better culture and, therefore, a higher profit margin as a natural byproduct.

Why then don't more companies and healthcare organizations place their primary focus on employees? Well, imagine having this conversation with the CEOs or CFOs at your local hospital. After explaining the People First framework to them, you are likely to hear something like, "Wait, you are telling me that if I invest in physician well-being and these ABCs of Self-Determination that my profit margin will actually increase?" They then look down at their balance sheet and add the cost of your initiatives directly to the expense column and say, "But when I add these changes to the balance sheet, they all end up in the expense category, which only increases our cost and drives our profit down! See? This could never work!"

Of course, I am being sarcastic, but the reality isn't that far off. Still, there might be some pundits out there who would say, "Jimmy,

---

22 Àine Cain, "Costco Workers Reveal 33 Things They'd Love to Tell Shoppers, but Can't," *Business Insider*, September 30, 2019, https://www.businessinsider.com/costco-membership-what-employees-want-to-say-2018-4#dont-make-assumptions-about-employees-happiness-19.

it feels like you are splitting hairs. If our target is profit where good culture is hopefully the byproduct, how is that different from focusing on people first where profit is the byproduct?" To them I would say that they have a lot to learn from New Zealand Flight 901 and from chasing two rabbits at once. Being even slightly off of our intended target matters more than we can appreciate in the long run. It may seem subtle, but as Simon Sinek points out, "When leaders are willing to prioritize trust over performance, performance almost always follows. However, when leaders have laser-focus on performance above all else, the culture inevitably suffers."

As leaders in medicine have focused on profit and performance above all else, our culture is failing. Like Flight 901, we are heading directly into Mount Erebus, and many leaders don't realize it. The clouds are about to break. We are about to descend. The alarms are going off. And there will be countless burned-out healthcare workers as a result. That is, unless physicians on the front line decide to fight back. This is our watershed moment in medicine. We can allow profit-first models to continue, which will result in burnout. Or, we can force this system to focus on people first, which will create self-determined physicians.

# PART 2

# THE INDIVIDUAL PHYSICIAN FIGHT

CHANGE IS COMING, whether healthcare likes it or not. For organizations that create great workplace cultures, this will result in a world in which medical professionals show up to work each day engaged, intrinsically motivated, and fulfilled. This will result in the profit margin healthcare organizations need to accomplish their missions. Yet, this will only happen if people are prioritized over profit.

However, I also realize that many healthcare organizations are reluctant to change, and this will inevitably leave a large portion of burned-out physicians working in cultures on the left side of the Healthcare Culture Continuum. That is why the remainder of this book is meant to help burned-out doctors understand the individual obstacles they face and to help them defeat burnout so that they create a life they love. Even if the hospitals and clinics where you work fail to do so. The purpose of this book, then, is to someday no longer be needed, because that will mean that we have fixed (or at least made meaningful progress toward fixing) the culture of medicine that burns out so many medical professionals.

From here on out, this book will be about helping you to become self-determined like Nelson Mandela, Maya Angelou, and so many others. And to teach you the tools that I've learned in helping hundreds of doctors defeat their own burnout and create a life they love inside (and outside) of medicine. Because only when we have enough self-determined physicians will we really be able to stand up, have a voice, and demand the changes we all know medicine needs. To shift the Healthcare Culture Continuum firmly to the right. This is the shared vision of self-determined physicians. If we band together, we will be a strong and mighty force that must be reckoned with, and while this journey is not for the faint of heart, I can tell you it is 100% worth it. So, if you are ready to learn how to experience self-determination for yourself, let's take a look at why so many doctors feel helpless in the first place.

# CHAPTER 4

# Learned Helplessness

"We have met the enemy, and the enemy is us."
—Walt Kelly

IN 1967, MARTIN Seligman, an American psychologist, performed a two-part experiment on German shepherds. In Seligman's study, there were three groups of dogs. In part one of this experiment, all three groups of dogs were placed in harnesses. Here is how they were broken up:

- Group 1 dogs were put in a harness and later released. This was the control group. Nothing happened to them while placed in the harness.
- Group 2 dogs were administered an electric shock through their harness that they could stop by pressing on a lever located in the box in which they were placed.
- Group 3 dogs received the same shocks as Group 2 dogs, but their lever did not work. When they pressed it, they continued to get shocked.

As expected, no change was noted in the Group 1 dogs. The dogs in Group 2 learned that their shocks could be stopped when they took action by pressing the lever. But for the dogs in Group 3, they quickly learned that there was nothing they could do about getting shocked. In other words, they learned that they had no autonomy.

In part two of the experiment, the German shepherds were placed into a different box that had a small divider on the ground that all of the dogs could easily jump over. One side of Seligman's research box shocked the dogs. The other side did not. Between the two sections was the small divider. All of the dogs were first placed in the side that would administer a shock. If the dog remained on the side of the box where they were initially placed, they would continue to be shocked. If they jumped over the divider to the other side of the box, the shocks would stop.

What happened next proved enlightening. After being placed in this box, the dogs in the first two groups did what we would expect. They realized that by jumping over the small divider, they could end their discomfort. So, that's exactly what they did. They felt pain, took control, jumped over the divider, and stopped getting shocked.

That's not what happened in Group 3, however. Remember, this is the group that learned they had no control or autonomy in their situation. Their lever didn't work in part 1 of the experiment. So, they felt that there was nothing they could do to stop their discomfort. When placed into Seligman's second box, the Group 3 dogs did not jump over the small barrier to the other side. In fact, 66%, or two out of three of the dogs in Group 3, laid down and did nothing. Except whine. All they had to do was jump over the small divider to the other side of the box, and most of them didn't even try to end their discomfort.

Seligman's experiment on German shepherds would lead to the term "learned helplessness." Oxford dictionary defines learned helplessness as "a condition in which a person suffers from a sense of powerlessness, arising from a traumatic event or persistent failure to succeed." Learned helplessness is the same phenomenon that happens in abusive relationships where an abused spouse stays because they have learned that there is nothing they can do to stop the abuse.

It is also the same phenomenon that many burned-out physicians experience when they have their personal and professional autonomy continually taken away from them. At first, doctors might try to fix their situation by going part-time, cutting back, or asking an administrator for the change they need. This is their attempt to press the lever in the box like the Group 3 German shepherds. After their suggestions or changes don't work, doctors realize that their lever is broken. That is when burned-out doctors succumb to the same learned helplessness the Group 3 German shepherds experienced. Many doctors then stay in a culture of burnout on the left side of the Healthcare Culture Continuum. They feel powerless. So, they lie down in their box of burnout because they feel powerless.

Perhaps this explains why one of the most common phrases I hear burned-out doctors say about the state of medicine is "that's just the way it is" or "this is the way we have always done it" as if there is nothing that can be done about changing the culture of medicine. Instead of continuing to fight for the change that we all know the culture of medicine needs, Group 3 doctors simply lie down and get shocked. As both a German shepherd owner and a physician, when I think about Seligman's research and findings, it makes me sad.

## DEFEATING LEARNED HELPLESSNESS

Fortunately, doctors are not German shepherds. Humans have the ability to defeat their learned helplessness because it is a type of conditioning. Learned helplessness is a paradigm that we have accepted. Unlike the German shepherds in the experiment, we know that people can reverse conditioning through unlearning our previous ways of thinking and relearning new ways. This is the work we do in coaching. Burned-out physicians can examine whether their thoughts are valid or helpful. Are doctors really trapped or stuck in medicine? Do they really not belong with the other doctors in Group 1 and Group 2? Is it really true that there is nothing that they can do?

Separating our story from the facts is an important exercise that I often employ when coaching a client. I call this being a "curious skeptic." Skeptical because my job is to avoid believing anything that my client's mind offers up. Clients already believe their own story, and it isn't producing the results they want in their life. In order to help burned-out doctors, coaches need to be curious and ask questions about whether their client's story is serving them. In other words, the most helpful coaches will help poke holes in the client's story so that we can see more clearly. When an objective third party allows you to see that your paradigm is not serving you, the scales can fall off your blinded eyes and you can finally see that your learned helplessness is a choice.

When burned-out doctors refuse to believe their story of learned helplessness, that is when the real work begins. That is when doctors realize that they aren't nearly as helpless as they thought. This is the first step in reclaiming personal and professional autonomy. Just as it took repeated abuses by the system to learn helplessness, unlearning that narrative and replacing it with another paradigm or perspective takes iterative practice, too. Yet, if we practice, practice really can make perfect.

## PRACTICE MAKES PERFECT

We know that practice can make perfect. We have seen this happen many times in our life. For example, none of us were born knowing how to drive a car (*except Lewis Hamilton—that guy probably knew how to drive from birth*). I remember the first time I drove my first car, a maroon-and-black 1989 Ford Mustang. I had to think about every single step, from turning the key to fire the ignition, putting the shifter in reverse, and then shifting gears again to drive away after narrowly missing my mailbox in our driveway. Then, I learned to step on the gas, flip the blinker, shift lanes, and so on. Honestly, I think my dad still has PTSD from me rolling through some stop signs and driving on the wrong side of the road when I first started driving. None of it was natural to me.

Yet, I now frequently drive home on autopilot without really remembering the drive because it has become such an automatic experience. In other words, I have conditioned myself to learn how to drive. I have taken what was previously a very intentional and laborious process and made it easy and automatic. Practice really has made perfect. I bet many of you can relate to this experience, too, even if you never drove on the wrong side of the road!

This ideology that practice makes perfect is captured in the work of Daniel Kahneman and Amos Tversky, two Israeli psychologists who spent their careers studying decision-making. After many years perfecting their work, Kahneman and Tversky created a name for the systems we use for thinking. The slow, methodical, and intentional decision-making process like the one we used when we first learned how to drive is called System 2. Other examples of System 2 thinking include asking someone to add 436 + 259, parallel parking a car in a tight space, or writing a thesis for a PhD. For most, the decisions involved in these activities require slow and deliberate thinking. We cannot do it automatically.

Other decisions or thought processes are fast, intuitive, and automatic. For example, if I asked you to finish the phrase, "War and..." you will likely say "peace"; if I ask you to add 2 + 2, you'll without hesitation say, "4"; and if I asked you to shift lanes while on the interstate, it would happen fluidly. Kahneman and Tversky labeled these fluid and automatic thought processes System 1.

Fortunately, like learning how to drive or memorizing a multiplication table, we can transition many processes from a System 2

to a System 1 style of thinking. With practice, we can make a previously laborious process automatic. This can happen with learned
helplessness as well. We can learn how to decondition that automatic System 1 thought that "we have no control." We don't have
to believe our options are limited or that there is nothing we can do
about the aspects of our plight in medicine.

Then, we can choose to replace that automatic System 1 thought
by recognizing that we always have a choice. Realizing that like Nelson Mandela showed us, it is up to us what we do with our thoughts.
That we do not have to say yes to the checkboxes placed in front
of us. The online modules, charting demands, and the like are all a
choice. Even walking into work—as strange as it sounds—is a volun-
tary choice. There is no invisible force making choices for us.

Yet, for me, it didn't feel like a choice in the midst of my burnout
when I was getting home late. Again. When I had to miss my kid's
T-ball game or gymnastics practice. When I brought work home
because I couldn't get it done while I was at the hospital. When
there was another online module or checklist to complete. Or when
the medical billers told me that I needed to attest to CPR after I lost
a patient on the surgical table. Simply put, I didn't feel like the captain of my own ship. However, that was about to change. In order to
decondition my learned helplessness and become the master of my
thoughts, first I needed to learn how my thoughts had become the
master of me.

# CHAPTER 5

# When Our Thoughts Master Us

"You are today where your thoughts have brought you;
you will be tomorrow where your thoughts take you."
—James Allen

AN AMERICAN INVESTMENT banker was taking a much-needed vacation in a small coastal Mexican village when a small boat with just one fisherman docked. The boat had several large, fresh fish in it. The investment banker was impressed by the quality of the fish and asked the Mexican how long it took to catch them. The Mexican replied, "Only a little while."

The banker then asked why he didn't stay out longer and catch more fish. The Mexican fisherman replied that he had enough to support his family's immediate needs. The American then asked, "But what do you do with the rest of your time?"

"I sleep late, fish a little, play with my children, take siesta with my wife, stroll into the village each evening where I sip wine and play guitar with my amigos," the Mexican fisherman replied. "I have a full and busy life, señor."

The investment banker scoffed. "I am an Ivy League MBA, and I could help you. You could spend more time fishing and with the proceeds, buy a bigger boat. And with the proceeds from the bigger boat, you could buy several boats, until eventually, you would have a whole fleet of fishing boats. Instead of selling your catch to the middleman, you could sell directly to the processor, eventually opening your own cannery. You could control the product, processing and distribution."

Then he added: "Of course, you would need to leave this small coastal fishing village and move to Mexico City where you would run your growing enterprise."

The Mexican fisherman asked, "But señor, how long will this all take?"

To which the American replied: "Fifteen to twenty years."

"But what then?" asked the Mexican.

The American laughed and said, "That's the best part. When the time is right, you would announce an IPO and sell your company stock to the public and become very rich. You could make millions."

"Millions, señor? Then what?"

To which the investment banker replied, "Then you would retire. You could move to a small coastal fishing village where you would sleep late, fish a little, play with your kids, take siesta with your wife, stroll to the village in the evenings where you could sip wine and play your guitar with your amigos."

How powerful is this well-known parable?[23] The main difference in this story, of course, is the perspective on what "should" be done

---

23  Faisal Jamshaid, "What You Can Learn From a Mexican Fisherman," *Medium*, June 7, 2020, https://medium.com/life-lemons/what-you-can -learn-from-a-mexican-fisherman-a8334882204c.

with the fish. The Mexican fisherman holds a people-over-profit focus, where he aims to catch enough fish to live a life full of autonomy and belonging. The American investment banker, on the other hand, shares the profit-over-people focus that many of our healthcare organizations have, where the primary focus is on money so that someday we can live the life we want. No margin, no mission. Sound familiar?

Isn't it amazing the difference a single thought can make? During my coaching certification process, we were taught that there are no "true" thoughts or "false" thoughts. Instead, there are only thoughts that serve us and thoughts that don't. Though I believe that there are some absolute truths in this world (for example, genocide is wrong), the lesson remains. Thoughts can either serve us and lead to results we want, or they can hinder us in our journey to becoming self-determined physicians. The sooner we can discover and drive out the unintentional thoughts that do not serve us, the sooner we will be able to shift our continuum toward becoming self-determined. Regardless of what our healthcare organizations do.

Jon Acuff, the author of *Soundtracks: The Surprising Solution to Overthinking,* has a similar take to what is taught in coaching school. Acuff calls our firmly entrenched thoughts a soundtrack. These soundtracks, he argues, can either serve us or work against us. You may be curious how you can tell if a thought is serving you or not. When we aren't sure if a particular thought is helpful or not, Acuff encourages us to ask three questions to sort it out.

First—"Is it true?" With this question, Acuff is asking us to realize what we have already discussed. Is the narrative, paradigm, or story that we are telling ourselves really a "fact?" Or, is it just a thought, paradigm, or perspective about our external situation?

Second—"Is the thought helpful?" Is our thought allowing us to improve our autonomy, sense of belonging, or perceived competence? Is it helping us become self-determined? If not, maybe this broken soundtrack should go the way of the dodo bird.

The third and final question Acuff proposes is the hardest for most physicians because so many doctors are their own worst critic. Acuff's third question, "Is it kind?" helps us determine if we are showing the sort of compassion to ourselves that we would show to someone else. Does our thought give us a deeper sense of purpose and belonging? Is it helping us get to where we want to go? Or is the thought beating us down?

Acuff's three questions help us catch our errant ways of thinking. In coaching terms, these questions allow us to get rid of thoughts that aren't serving us. While we cannot control the institutions of medicine that create cultures of burned-out physicians, we must realize that we are not helpless Group 3 German Shepherds, either. In our search for autonomy, the goal is to become the master of your thoughts. Yet, before we can discuss how to become the master of our thoughts (the focus of Part 3 of this book), we must first learn how our thoughts have a tendency to master us. These errant ways of thinking are called cognitive distortions.

## COGNITIVE DISTORTIONS

Cognitive distortions are described as "tendencies or patterns of thinking or believing" that are "false or inaccurate" and that "have the potential to cause psychological damage."[24]

You can think of cognitive distortions as thoughts dressed in sheep's clothing, who seem innocent but are more like ravenous wolves stealing our ABCs of self-determination. While they seem innocuous, these distorted thoughts have a profound impact on our life. Below are five of the most common cognitive distortions that

---

24   Courtney Ackerman, "Cognitive Distortions: 22 Examples & Worksheets," PositivePsychology.com, https://positivepsychology.com/cognitive-distortions/.

I've seen plague the physicians we coach. As you read about them, I want you to be aware of how and where these disruptive thoughts may exist in your life. When they come up, this should raise a red flag that you may be heading more toward burnout on the culture continuum than you are toward self-determination.

## 1. All-or-Nothing (a.k.a. Dichotomous Thinking)

My favorite characters in movies are neither completely good nor completely bad. We see them rise to great heights and fall to great depths. A great example of this is Professor Snape from *Harry Potter*, who is presumed to be evil for the majority of the series. Yet, in the end, he proves to have the potential for good as well. His character is never wholly good or wholly bad. He lives in the murky in-between. In the land of gray. Just like us.

Yet, many of us have a tendency to fall prey to black-and-white thinking. Particularly when things are not going well. We have a tendency to think that things are entirely good or entirely bad. Maybe your employer—while going through tough economic times—decided to take away your 401(k) matching. Perhaps they make you pick up extra shifts, see more patients, or work longer hours without paying you more. For some, it might be a transition to a new EMR that turns out to be hard to learn, unsafe, or makes it more challenging to care for patients.

All of these situations seem negative. They may lead you to say things like "This job is terrible" or "Clearly, none of the bean counters upstairs care about what their decisions do to me." These statements fail to acknowledge the aspects of our job that may be good, and they destroy our sense of belonging in our medical offices and hospitals. Devoid of shades of gray, this is called black-and-white, or dichotomous, thinking.

Dichotomous thinking is similar to the splitting phenomenon seen in borderline personality disorder (BPD), where these patients see people as either all-good or all-bad. Unlike BPD patients, however, this is not a personality trait, but a temporary thought error that can be noticed and corrected, like a red flag. Some of the words we might use when we are trapped in dichotomous thinking include words like "always," "never," or "every time." This shows an inability to see shades of gray, and it is a sign that we may be stuck in an all-or-nothing cognitive distortion.

When we catastrophize through dichotomous thinking, we miss that there may be facets of our situation that are still good or even great. We may still enjoy working with our coworkers, love our patient population, or feel productive and full of purpose at the end of most workdays. Yet, when our focus is placed squarely on the negative aspects of our job as if they are the only parts that exist, this mindset forces us more toward burnout and distances us from becoming self-determined physicians.

Once, I had a client who was a burned-out pediatrician, Jonah. Jonah's boss wasn't supportive, and he felt that the job had changed for the worse. So, Jonah started looking for a new job when he joined our coaching program. I asked Jonah what the biggest issue seemed to be. He said, "Well, it's these terrible meetings where nothing gets done. They are completely pointless. In times past, we didn't even have these meetings. Now, I have to go, and it is just miserable!"

Being the curious skeptic, I pushed Jonah further on the facts. It turned out that these meetings happened once or twice per month for one hour each. I asked him what he thought about the rest of the job. After taking a moment to reflect, Jonah said, "You know? I actually love the rest of my job. I've always loved being a doctor." When I pointed out Jonah's black-and-white language about the job due to two hours of meetings per month while he ignored the other, enjoyable 98% of the time he spent performing patient care, Jonah realized he had fallen into dichotomous thinking. None of us are immune to this all-or-nothing cognitive distortion, but being aware that it exists is half the battle.

The take-home point is this: while sometimes circumstances can be "wholly good" or "wholly bad," most of the time there are shades of gray. Having a fair look at the situation and reminding ourselves of both the good and bad that exist is often enough to send us toward the sense of belonging and deeper purpose we all desire. It is a helpful exercise that fosters gratitude instead of groveling.

## 2. Overgeneralization and Shame

When I was an intern on my emergency medicine rotation, we had an elderly patient who was on warfarin with an INR of ~3.5. She was septic and needed a central line for access so that we could run vasopressors. At this point in my career, I had built central lines up to be this critical procedure that ought to be in the wheelhouse of any good anesthesiologist. You could either place a central line in five minutes, or you were a bad anesthesiologist. That's the story I created anyway. Talk about some all-or-nothing thinking.

On this particular shift, I stayed well after midnight when my shift ended to attempt my first central line on this septic patient with a supratherapeutic INR. During the procedure, all was going well until I started to take the wire out. As I removed the wire, I unintentionally pulled the whole shebang out of the patient (including the wire and the central line). With an INR over 3, a hematoma immediately began to form. My face flushed, my palms began to sweat, and I felt like a complete idiot. I looked at my upper-level emergency medicine resident like a young child would when they make a grave mistake, hoping for some assurance. Something like "That's okay, no big deal, buddy!" Instead my upper-level resident said, "Well, you'll never do *that* again. Hold pressure; I'll put my gown on." I was mortified.

That night, I went home and couldn't sleep for hours. Why? Because, in my mind, placing a central line was something any anesthesia resident worth a lick of salt should easily be able to accomplish. I started thinking things like *"I can't believe I did that...I'm such a failure. I am going to be a terrible anesthesiologist."* Lacking perspective, I had taken a single moment and amplified it into who and what I was. One botched procedure and I was, therefore, a failure and a terrible anesthesiologist-in-training. This cognitive distortion where we take a single incident and make it mean much more is called overgeneralization, and it often leads to shame.

Shame is deadly in our work to become self-determined physicians. And overgeneralization can lead to a full-fledged shame suck fest that attacks any sense of belonging we might have. In order to understand this better, we need to have a full grasp on shame.

One of my favorite authors is Brené Brown—a leading shame researcher, social worker, and speaker. I've yet to find a book by the good Dr. Brown that I didn't love. To date, Brown provides the best explanation I've seen on the difference between guilt and shame. She explains that guilt is a feeling that happens when we make a mistake. Shame is a feeling we experience when something goes wrong and we feel like *we* are the mistake. Guilt is a focus on the mistake. Shame is a focus on our identity. Brown puts it this way, "Guilt is 'I did something bad,' whereas shame is 'I am bad.'" Overgeneralization does not usually lead to guilt. It often leads to shame. That is why it is such a dangerous cognitive distortion.

If I only felt guilt about how the central line had gone in my septic patient, I would have said, "That was stupid" and shook it off the same way I do when I cannot remember where I placed my keys. This is healthy. This sort of guilt often prompts us to improve the next time. Instead, my overgeneralization made the procedure mean something about my overall identity as a physician. It cut to my core and directly impacted my perceived competence—one of the three elements of a burned-out physician. I believed "I am a bad doctor." While guilt is something outside of us, shame is internal. After the central line, I adopted the identity that I was a failure who was destined to be a bad anesthesiologist. All because of one procedure. This is how powerful overgeneralization can be, if we let it.

From an outside vantage point, you may read that central-line story and realize my thinking was flawed and lacked perspective. You are right. But that didn't keep me from staying up for another three hours, unable to fall asleep that night. When you are trapped in a cognitive distortion, it requires you to either recognize it or have an objective third party like a counselor or coach point it out to you.

Overgeneralization can be directed both internally or to other people externally. While the internal version of overgeneralization can attack our sense of belonging and competence, the external iteration more readily attacks our sense of community and team. When overgeneralization is directed at others, it shifts our healthcare culture continuum toward bitterness and burnout.

For example, a client of ours named Harper once had a physician colleague with a penchant for showing up late. On the specific occasion we were discussing, Harper's partner at work was supposed to relieve her from her shift. Yet, they were late to show up. This had happened before. It really bothered Harper. So, she brought it to a group coaching call to get some outside perspective. Due to these prior situations, Harper believed that her partner was selfish and did not respect her time. She felt that her colleague had a total lack of respect for other people. Therefore, Harper took this partner's penchant for being late and made it mean that her colleague was a terrible partner in practice. What Harper was doing was overgeneralizing a partner showing up late for work and making it mean that they were a bad partner. This was despite the fact that her partner was otherwise great to work with. (Not to mention, Harper had never discussed her concerns with her colleague). You can imagine what Harper's overgeneralization did to the teamwork, camaraderie, and shared sense of belonging in that group. The community was under attack.

In order to combat the cognitive distortion of overgeneralization, it requires a fresh perspective. It requires us to take in a broader picture. Does that one patient review, medical malpractice suit, or situation really define who we are as a physician? When you notice that you are in a fight against overgeneralization, I'd encourage you to break out the pen and paper. Fold the paper in half (hot-dog style), and then write down your current thought on one side (I prefer the left since "sinister" in Latin means "on the left side"). On the right side, write down all of your experiences that fly directly in the face of this boldfaced and sinister lie you are currently telling yourself.

For example, if I had done this exercise as an intern following my central-line escapade, I could have written down "I am a bad doctor because I botched a central line" on the sinister side of my paper. On the right side, I could have written down other thoughts that disproved my being a bad doctor. Thoughts like the following:

- My clinical evaluations say that I am doing pretty well. Above average, in fact.
- No one has ever pulled me aside and told me I am doing a bad job.
- I placed two ultrasound-guided IVs the other day without any problem.
- I am only an intern...There is a lot to learn from this experience.
- Being a good doctor involves more than placing central lines.

We must remember that our value (and anyone else's value, too) is much more than a single bad day or decision. We are worthy and enough, just the way we are. Right now. And granting this same view to other people in our life goes a long way toward creating a self-determined culture where we live and work.

## 3. "Should" Statements

There may not be a more pervasive, yet harmful, word in the English language than "should." If you don't believe me, watch out for this word the rest of the day and notice how it feels when it comes up. I *should* call that person back, even though I don't want to talk to them. I *should* get that paper or project done, even though I have bigger fish to fry right now. I *should* stay quiet and be respectful, even though no one else is standing up for what is right. I *should* not have missed that read, diagnosis, or call...even though many other colleagues likely would have done the same. Other words people sometimes use in place of should include "ought," "need to," or "have to." I "should" call the person back is the same as I ought to call them back, I need to call them back, and I have to call them back.

Let me give you an example of the power of this cognitive distortion. The most painful mistake I've made to date as an attending physician actually wasn't with a patient. It was with a resident during a lecture. For some background on this, I should mention (*man, that word really does sneak up on us, doesn't it?*) that I care very deeply about diversity and inclusion and, in particular, civil rights for brown and black people. This passion started when my friend Nick, a Black pastor in the AME church, forever changed my life and perspective when we became friends.

Nick would say things like, "Jimmy, when you were in high school and you went into the cafeteria, did it ever cross your mind, 'Huh, I wonder why all the Black kids sit by themselves? Why don't they come sit with us?"

To which I replied, "Yeah, Nick, I did think that in high school."

Then, Nick asked, "Did it ever cross your mind, 'I wonder why all the white kids sit with themselves? Why don't the white kids go sit with the black kids?" If I was being honest, that thought had never crossed my mind as a high school student. Ever. Slowly, but surely, Nick chipped away at the prejudice that I didn't know was there.

Nick had this way of showing how deep my implicit bias as a white male ran, while also showing me grace and compassion. I needed to be shown the error of my ways, and Nick was patient enough to help me do that. Many conversations with Nick were like the first time I saw an IMAX 3D movie in 2009. The movie was Steven Spielberg's *Avatar*. The way the characters jumped off the screen and into your field of vision was so real. It was like being in the movie with the characters, like a fly on the wall. Because of that immersive experience, I have never been able to watch the movie *Avatar* on a regular 2D TV. I simply cannot see the movie any other way. Nick had the same impact on me. I now notice systemic and systematic racial injustice everywhere and stand firmly and openly against it.

The reason I tell you this background is because the low point in my career as an attending physician happened when I called one of our Black residents in our residency program by the name of another Black resident during a lecture. I didn't immediately recognize my mistake. It was after the lecture that it suddenly dawned on me that I had called our resident the wrong name. With the above background in mind, I was absolutely mortified. That's when the "should" statements started. "Great, I'm just another example of some privileged white male attending physician treating someone of color as if they are all the same. I *should not* have done that. What an idiot. Our resident is never going to forgive me."

With my inner critic headed into overdrive, I went to the resident break room where our residents often hang out. I wanted to explain how unforgivable my mistake had been and that I was truly sorry for being so insensitive. Unfortunately, the resident I was looking for wasn't there. Instead, I spent the next forty-eight hours writing, sending, and then rereading my apology email to this resident while I waited for a response. When that resident didn't respond for the next forty-eight hours, my brain had all the information it needed to crucify my self-worth and any sense of belonging as a flag-bearing member of the anti-racist community. Based on my values, I had completely failed in one of the most unacceptable ways imaginable. Finally, our resident responded and provided me with the same grace and forgiveness that Nick often did in our conversations when I put my foot in my mouth.

That didn't stop me from tormenting myself during those forty-eight hours while awaiting a response. The problem with "should" statements is that they imply that there is a right or wrong way to do something. And that if we don't do it that way, we have made a huge mistake. "Should" statements are statements of criticism about who we are and what we have or haven't done. When I made the aforementioned mistake with our resident's name, I did something that caused cognitive dissonance for someone who opposes all forms of racism whether individual or systemic.

As with other cognitive distortions, "should" statements can be both internal or external. We all have an idea of what a good spouse, parent, teacher, friend, or physician "should" look like. As our everyday thoughts, words, and experiences differ from the ideals and values we hold, "should" statements provide the same cognitive dissonance I experienced during the forty-eight hours after my lecture.

*As an aside, the resident in the story above didn't check their email for two days, which is why it took forty-eight hours to hear back. They were incredibly gracious with my mistake. Even still, I apologized approximately 172 times.*

## Internal "Should" Statements

As mentioned, "should" statements can be both internal and external. Jasmine was a client of ours in ACE who felt like she was in a catch-22, being both a mom and a physician. When Jasmine was on inpatient call for the week, she experienced longer hours that caused her to be away from her family more than usual. This would result in lots of tears from her children as they clung to her leg begging her not to leave. When this happened, she felt like she was damned if she stayed and damned if she didn't. Regardless of what she decided, Jasmine wasn't doing what a "good mom" or a "good doctor" *should* do. Either way, her sense of belonging at home or at work was threatened.

This situation produced internal conflict each time she was on call. One narrative told her that a good mom would be around her kids more. Yet, Jasmine also realized that if she stayed, she would experience the inner-self-critic that told her that she would be wasting her skill, education, and training if she didn't maximize her potential to help others as a physician. Because Jasmine was on call in regular intervals, she began to dread her weeks on call. Not because the shifts were terrible, but because the cognitive dissonance caused by her "should" statements was so powerful.

Internal "should" statements imply that if we don't do something we feel we ought to do, we are not living up to our moral standard. I often call this phenomenon "shoulding ourselves into shame." Jasmine was choosing to believe that when she left the house for work while her kids were begging her to stay, it was a sign that she was not a good mom. A good mom should be around her kids as much as possible, right? Being the curious skeptic, I asked Jasmine if she ever had a time when she was around the kids a lot (say, on vacation) where they still didn't want her to leave (perhaps while going to have lunch with a friend or taking a trip to the store). I asked her to recall a situation where her kids said, "Mommy, we don't want you to leave," even when they were consistently getting time with her. After thinking about it, Jasmine realized it happened the last time she was on vacation with her family at the beach. Suddenly, she realized that her kids asking her not to leave wasn't a sign that she was a bad mom. In fact, it was proof that her kids loved and adored her. And, no matter how much time Jasmine spent with her family, her kids would always want more.

So why did Jasmine feel so bad? Because her "should" statements were malignant. In the end, she realized that she is the one who gets to decide what a good doctor and a good mom looks like. These "should" statements were not serving her. When her kids clung to her leg the next time she was leaving the house while on call, Jasmine shifted her perspective toward self-determination. Her kids asking her to stay was evidence that she was indeed a fantastic mom and physician who did exactly what she "should" be doing. She felt like she belonged both at home and at work. In the end, Jasmine felt like she was both a good mom and a good doctor, which she was, and is.

## External "Should" Statements

Odds are, unless you live and work in isolation, you likely have an unwritten how-to guide. These how-to guides describe how you expect your husband, wife, partner, child, parent, sibling, or colleague to act. As I mentioned, these guides are not publicly written documents to which people can refer. *Uh, excuse me, ma'am, can you please refer to section 3-2 for how to appropriately address me when I greet you at work?* Naturally, this lack of explicit expectations can lead to a lot of resentment and bitterness toward the people in our life when they don't act according to our unwritten rule book.

For example, let's say that I've picked my kids up from school, and I am now about to cook dinner for my family. My three kids, who are all under the age of eleven, are running around like buffoons—likely playing "horsey" where one of my kids pulls the other using a blanket until one of them collides with a hard object like the arm of the couch. Or the floor. Or the chair that my third kid intentionally put in the way to cause mayhem. That's when the screaming and crying starts. I'm still trying to cook dinner throughout all of this, of course.

So, when my wife, Kristen, gets home from work, I may expect her to drop everything she is doing to watch the kids so that I can cook dinner. On the other hand, Kristen may expect me to give her some time to decompress. She needs to collect her thoughts and take a moment after a long day at work. Because neither of us have talked about our expectations—and yet we both still have them—we will both have thoughts about what the other person "should" be doing.

My thought may be that *she should be helping me with the kids.* This produces feelings of anger and resentment if she doesn't. From this place, I may snap at Kristen when she asks what we are having for dinner as I see her checking her phone. *I don't recommend this course of action for any spouses out there, by the way.* Then we fight. This isn't fair to Kristen. She has no idea what I expect from her, and Kristen is a grown woman. She gets to do whatever she wants regardless of what my expectations are, and if I slowed down to think about it, that is actually what I want. Autonomy is one of the core tenets of self-determination that we have discussed at length in this book. If I love my wife, I don't want to control her. And I certainly don't want her controlling me.

The kids going crazy at dinnertime wasn't caused by Kristen's unwillingness to help or by my unwillingness to let her decompress. It was caused by unstated expectations that create external "should" statements about what we think the other should be doing. In other words, it isn't caused by the circumstances of the situations; it is caused by the cognitive distortions we have about them. And, if unchecked, these external "should" statements have the propensity to attack our sense of belonging.

## 4. Believing You Need to Be Right

Most physicians are perfectionists, which can cause us to fall into the unfortunate trap of needing to be "right." This cognitive distortion serves as a red herring in many conversations and coaching calls. When the focus of our argument is on being "right" and the other person being "wrong," we have likely lost focus on what is most important—our need to feel like valued members of a team who share a common purpose. When we are more concerned with being right than about the team members in our conversations, it is easy for people to feel disrespected, unappreciated, and like they are no longer a valued member of the team. We are attacking their self-determination.

This happens most often in what can be called crucial conversations. In a book by the same name,[25] the authors state that crucial conversations have three key elements. Crucial conversations are:

1. **Emotionally charged**—crucial conversations occur where you can feel your blood boiling, tensions rising, or you are otherwise emotional.
2. **A difference of opinions**—the parties involved do not agree on the matter at hand.
3. **High-stakes conversations**—the outcome of the conversation matters greatly to those involved.

As an example, say you are having a conversation with your partner about whether you "should" (note the "should" statement already puts this conversation into emotionally charged territory) put your kid into private school or public school. You feel that they should go to public school, while your partner feels that a private school would be best. This may start out as a friendly conversation, but it has all three components of a crucial conversation. It involves your children and is, therefore, a high-stakes conversation that also involves a difference of opinion and can easily become emotionally charged.

The conversation may start with the mutual goal of doing what is best for your child. However, at some point, the conversation devolves into which type of schooling is more likely to result in admission to college. Or maybe on what kind of school a doctor's child "should" attend. This is when tensions rise, and it is also when your focus has the potential to shift from doing what is best for your child to "winning" the argument. Perhaps one of you went to public

---

25  Joseph Grenny et al., Crucial Conversations: Tools for Talking When Stakes Are High, 3rd ed. (New York: McGraw-Hill, 2022).

school, and the other attended a private school. You both think you turned out fine. Isn't that proof enough? Your focus has shifted from loving your partner and hearing their point of view to winning at all costs. You have entered into the cognitive distortion of believing you always need to be right.

The same errant thought process commonly happens in the operating room (OR), too. In the OR, there are multiple members of the team, which means that there are differences of opinion when a case gets delayed as to why a patient didn't make it to the operating room on time. Was the patient late to arrive? Did the check-in process malfunction? Were the preoperative nurses slow? Was it an IV access problem? Was it anesthesia? *For those that don't work in an operating room, the answer is that it is always anesthesia's fault—we seem to be the universal scapegoat in operating rooms around the world, but I digress.* We cannot change the past, and it is not about being right or wrong. Yet, the OR delay conversation usually devolves into a blame game. This proves to be entirely unhelpful for the current patient or for improving the process for the next.

Fortunately, there is a better way. The moment that we are able to transition from the "right/wrong" mentality to asking questions like "What is the goal here?" we can remember the ultimate reason for having the conversation in the first place. It isn't about being on the winning side in the fight to determine where our kid goes to school or to figure out who is to blame for the ten minute delay in getting the patient to the operating room. Instead, the focus is on our kid getting a solid and supportive education or on fixing the systematic issues that might have led to the delay without pointing fingers at individuals.

In addition to all of this, of course, we must remember that everyone has an innate need to belong to their community, and harsh words that result from the need to always be right often work directly counter to fostering a culture where people feel valued, heard, and appreciated. As Brené Brown often says, maybe our focus ought to be on *"getting* it right, not *being* right." Shifting our focus toward *how* we have a conversation so that people feel valued and respected is infinitely more important than being right. As my favorite quote from Maya Angelou says, "People will forget what you said, people will forget what you did, but people will never forget how you made them feel."

## A FINAL WORD

In the first part of this book, we have discussed a lot of the problems that plague both the healthcare institutions where we work and also the individual physician. We have touched on arrival fallacies, victim mindsets, burnout, and learned helplessness, and we've briefly introduced imposter syndrome. We discovered the ABCs (autonomy, belonging, and competence) of creating self-determined physicians. Our need for autonomy, belonging, and perceived competence are the ingredients we need to combat burnout.

Unfortunately, most of us recognize that while this all sounds well and good, many institutions where we work refuse to change the focus of their current profit-over-people model. There is a two-part mission here. The first is to fix the systematic issues that plague medicine. So, if you are a healthcare leader or administrator, go back and read the first half of this book.

The second part of this book's mission is to empower burned-out doctors to create a life they love, even if they are working in an institution that is reluctant to change its ways. If you are in that situation, don't worry. The rest of this book is written specifically to help you reclaim your autonomy, sense of belonging, and perceived competence, independent of what your organization or practice does. I'm not going to leave you with some pie-in-the-sky idealism. If the first two parts of this book defined "what" the problem is, the third and fourth parts will describe "how" to empower self-determined physicians working in broken systems, even if their workplaces refuse to shift their cultures to the right on the Healthcare Culture Continuum. If you are ready to put the work in, let's get to it!

# PART 3

# THE PROCESS

THE PHYSICIAN PHILOSOPHER was born in November 2017, five months after I finished my fellowship in Regional Anesthesia and Acute Pain Management at Wake Forest. The original tagline was "wealth & wellness" because I recognized—like many physicians— that financial independence and burnout are related topics. I hadn't fully formed the connection between Self-Determination Theory and burnout (yet), but even then I understood the role personal finance could play in helping burned-out doctors. At one point, the tagline of The Physician Philosopher website became "fighting burnout with financial independence." Thus, a personal finance blog for physicians was born.

Financial independence (or FI, which is what those in-the-know call it) can be defined as the point at which we no longer need to earn a paycheck to live our current lifestyle. In other words, FI is the point at which doctors can retire from medicine. It is financial freedom, and it is one way to create personal autonomy in your life. For many, this seems like the obvious answer to burnout. Having the ability to walk away can solve any problem, right? I thought so, too. That is why I spent the first two years of The Physician Philosopher teaching doctors about the powers of personal finance. I even published a book called *The Physician Philosopher's Guide to Personal Finance* in February 2019. The subtitle? *The 20% of Personal Finance Doctors Need to Know to Get 80% of the Results.*

I was—and still am—very proud of that book. It is an easy read for anyone who wants to learn how to get started on their personal finance journey. The irony, of course, is that while I helped other doctors fight their burnout with financial independence, I was quickly burning out myself. So, I did what I taught others to do. Kristen and I created a glide path to be able to retire in our mid-fortiess by saving a six-figure sum of money each year. Our FI goal was to get to ~$3.5 million, or approximately 25 times our annual expenses.

The problem was that my burnout was on a course to crush me long before we ever got to FI. This didn't deter me, though! I didn't bail on personal finance. Instead, I doubled down. I determined that if I could grow the bottom line at The Physician Philosopher, perhaps my online business could provide a quicker way to no longer be dependent on my clinical income as a physician. The more money The Physician Philosopher created, the less dependent I became on making money in medicine. This was a hybrid view of FI that combined the cash flow model used in real estate with the traditional "25 times your annual expense" model taught on many FI blogs. My focus on money as a tool to fight my burnout is well captured in a poem that I wrote when I was nearing rock bottom, called "The Truth Is." Here is where I was and where you might be, too, as you read or listen to this book:

The truth is, those of us in the trenches, we don't have a say.
And those in power are just trying to make it rain
dollar bills with their golden cuffs and parachute.
In their ivory towers, chasing metrics in a suit.
Screamin' from the burnout, begging for a change.
That won't happen, because our voice is out of range.

The truth is I'm sick of getting trapped in other people's trappings.
I used to care so much about what others thought was happening.
I wanted some approval...but now that doesn't matter.
Promotions, tenure, papers, it's all a bunch of chatter.

See, I wanna be a good doctor, but I hate having to choose
between being a good employee, a husband, and dad, too.
The truth is burnout can consume every ounce of what we love.
One less doctor, sister, mother, brother, father to adore.
The system must change; meditations and deep breathing
don't fix the problem, the morally injured are left seething.

It's time that we stand up, and demand what we deserve.
We can no longer be quiet; we're starting to strike a nerve.
The truth is the change can't happen, 'til those in power hear us.
"Be the change you want to see," that's what they tell us.

We write. We rap. We sing. We cry...
It all goes unheard 'til there's another death in the night.
Hard times and bad culture can change a man's mind.
More apathy, less compassion—we're breaking our design.

The truth is we don't have to be perfect; we don't have every answer,
but if this system doesn't change, it's going to grow like cancer.
Too young to be noticed, but too loud to be ignored.
They put doctors in the corner, and knock 'em to the floor.
Burned out by the thousands. But who's keeping score?
The truth is...we are. In our bank account. Until we can walk out
the door.

For a time, my focus on financial independence worked! I set
a goal in terms of annual cash flow, and as the business started to
take off, my bank account grew, too. As our nonclinical cash flow

increased, I was able to cut back in medicine, too. The only problem? Now, I was burning the candle at both ends at work and in my business, which led to a cataclysmic rate of burnout and a lack of work-life balance. This journey also pushed me further away from any sense of belonging that I had in medicine and proved to be another example that when we focus on profit over people (in this case, my business's profit over my own personal growth), it can prove to be highly problematic.

Yet, I am not alone in this experience. Many physicians try to get to their financial goals faster by earning more money through picking up extra shifts, working locums outside their main gig, staying in a job they hate to get to their financial goals faster, or starting a side gig while working full-time in medicine. With a primary focus on profit, you know what gets left behind? You and your well-being.

I want you to hear me loud and clear on this one. Money alone is not the answer. Money is a tool. It is the means to an end. Not the end itself. This is coming from someone who read, wrote, blogged, and podcasted about personal finance for physicians basically every single day for four years. Now, don't misread what I am saying. Money still plays an important role in personal autonomy. *I am still a self-proclaimed money nerd.* To this day, I still teach personal finance lectures to medical professionals, both in person for my fourth-year medical students at Wake Forest and online through my business at the Medical Degree Financial University (or MDFU—*yes, the FU to medicine pun is intended*). Financial freedom is also the reason that we created the *Money Meets Medicine* podcast to help doctors.

However, money is not the "end all, be all" that many would make it. It is one of many resources that allows us to get where we want to go in life. It is a part of reclaiming our personal autonomy, but it alone will not solve our burnout. In the People First Framework, personal autonomy is only responsible for 20% of our intended target. Money won't address your professional autonomy, help you feel like a valued member of the team, tie you to a deeper purpose, or help you with your perceived competence.

I have to admit that I had this backward for a long time. After creating enough financial freedom through The Physician Philosopher to allow me to go part-time in medicine and eventually leave medicine altogether if I wanted, I realized that—while this provided some short-term relief—there was still something missing. My focus on money proved to be another arrival fallacy. Financial independence was just a part of the recipe (personal autonomy), but I needed the other four ingredients of self-determination (professional autonomy, feeling valued as a team member, having a deeper purpose, and clinical confidence) if I was going to create the perfect recipe to becoming a self-determined physician.

I use the word recipe because creating a life you love is like baking a cake. Adding an ingredient at the wrong step or in the wrong order will not work. It is like adding the raw egg to your cake after you have already baked it instead of putting it into the mix before you pop it into the oven. Unless you like raw egg on top of an already-baked cake, this won't produce the end result you were looking for when you started, even though it involves the same ingredients. The ingredients have to be included in the proper amount, order, and timing to make a delicious cake.

It took going through this journey myself and then coaching hundreds of doctors to help them do the same before I realized that the order in which we use the tools matters. Just like the recipe for the cake requires a specific order and amount of ingredients, the tools we use to empower physicians ought to occur in a very specific order to help you become the hero of your story. Here is the three-part framework we use to help doctors become self-determined physicians all on their own. We call it The 3 Pillars to Physician Freedom.

You'll notice from the framework drawn above that, like the cake analogy, if you are missing an ingredient, then you are missing a key piece to the recipe. Without a mastery of your mindset—or the abil-

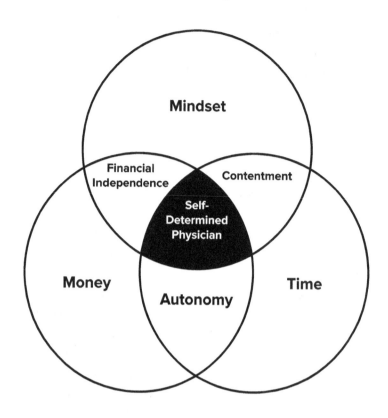

ity to control the internal narrative you have about your external circumstances like Nelson Mandela did on Robben Island—you will always lack contentment and likely suffer from imposter syndrome, learned helplessness, and/or a victim mindset. Without mastering money—creating a financial plan that will get you to financial freedom—you will always have to work and be a slave to your paycheck. In other words, you will not have personal autonomy. And without becoming a time management guru, you will live a life of hurry, where your personal and professional autonomy are under attack and where things that are highly important yet nonurgent (date nights, sleep, exercise, etc.) will get put on the back burner.

You might notice that in The 3 Pillars to Physician Freedom model, we have addressed how they help you obtain the autonomy and competence of the ABCs of self-determination. In addition to this framework, thousands of physicians are on the journey to ending personal and systemic burnout. We are on a journey to create a culture in medicine that not only allows physicians to enjoy their work, but that will also provide the best care to our patients. This is why studies show that group coaching and peer-to-peer conversations reduce burnout in physicians. Sharing our lived experience and knowing that we are not alone on this journey provides the deep sense of belonging that many of us lack in medicine.

This is the path, then. Mindset → Money → Life. And the order matters. Mastery over your mindset should come first in order to increase your autonomy and competence. Then, and only then, can money really be used properly as a tool to combat your burnout. And, finally, once you have the financial means to do so, you can begin to create the ideal life balance you want. Like learning to drive a car, we must first go to driving school to learn how to operate the car. This will happen when we master our mindset, which is the premise of the second half of this book. Then, we must learn how to put the fuel we need into the car in order to get to where we want to go (mastering your money, which is captured in *The Physician Philosopher's Guide to Personal Finance* and in content we teach on The Physician Philosopher. To learn more about these resources, you can visit thephysicianphilosopher.com/money). Once this is accomplished, only then can you determine how often and where you want to drive that car in order to best reflect your life's priorities.

As you start this journey, I want to share a letter I wrote to physicians (and to myself) when I was coming out of my burnout to remind myself that I was strong enough to endure anything that life could throw my way.

## You Have Always Been Strong

You were strong enough to get through weed-out classes in undergrad. You were strong enough to balance the extracurricular activities and clinical shadowing expected of you while crushing an eighteen- or twenty-one-hour semester. You were strong enough to say, "No, I have to study" when friends wanted to go out because you had a dream of becoming a doctor.

You were strong enough to pay for the applications, fight for the interviews, and earn your way into a matriculating medical school class. You were strong enough to defy the odds.

You were strong enough to withstand the rote memorization required in gross anatomy and biochemistry. You were strong enough to take on a seemingly insurmountable amount of debt.

You were strong enough to put on that white coat for the first time when it felt like the weight of the world's responsibilities now rested on your shoulders. You were strong enough to wear that same short white coat that labeled you a learner when you met your first patient on clinical rotations.

You were strong enough to say, "I know not."

You were strong enough to get through medical school and to match into residency. You were strong enough to face the long hours and sleepless nights. You were strong enough to put your head down, be a good soldier, and do what you were told. You were strong enough to miss weddings, funerals, and reunions.

You were strong enough to hold the hand of the first patient you ever lost. You were strong enough to tell her daughters of their loss—and strong enough to cry in front of them.

You were strong enough to come to work the day after because the next patient needed your help, too.

You were strong when you became an attending physician. You were strong when everyone looked to you to make the decision.

You were strong enough to deal with the imposter syndrome that you felt would consume you. You were strong when you were afraid you were a fraud. You were strong because you felt that strength was required of a good doctor.

You were strong the first time you made a difference or saved a life. You were strong when you gave the credit to the team. You were strong even when you received no credit at all.

You were strong because your patients needed you to be strong.

You were strong when you lost your autonomy for the first time along this journey to becoming a doctor. You were strong when your empathy began to fade.

You were strong when you felt overwhelmed by stress.

You were strong enough to deal with an insurance company dictating your patient's medical care. You were strong enough to deal with the administration's demand to increase your clinical workload and RVU production. You were strong enough to deal with the new electronic medical record system that was clearly meant for billing and not for patient care. You were strong enough to stand up for your patients when obstacles got in the way of their care. You were strong when you felt like a data-entry clerk.

You were strong the first time that you felt like quitting medicine. You were strong the first time you heard a fellow physician died by suicide. You were strong when you realized that the same doctor was a prior friend, classmate, and coworker.

You were strong even when you felt weak, depressed, and at the end of your rope.

You were strong when your family asked why you were coming home late. Again. You were strong enough to deal with the missed soccer games and recitals. You were strong when you got called back to the hospital—knowing that your kids would ask why they were the only ones who didn't have a parent at their school show.

You are still strong enough today. You are strong enough to talk with a therapist, coach, or counselor. You are strong enough to say no. You are strong enough to consider a change or to cut back your clinical hours at work. You are strong enough to know that you are valuable. You are strong enough to know you have options.

You are strong enough to realize that you are the master of your thoughts, feelings, actions, and results. You are strong enough to realize that once you've done the work, you can change your circumstances, if needed.

You are strong enough to know that you should not have to choose between being a good doctor, spouse, and parent. You are strong enough today to realize that asking for help isn't a sign of weakness. It is a sign of strength. You are strong enough to realize that you cannot do this on your own. You are strong enough to know that open and honest transparency will help fix this problem.

You are strong enough to know that we need strong doctors just like you.

* * *

If you are ready to join this community of strong doctors and fight back even when medicine won't fight for you, then it is time to get to work. It is time to start mastering your thoughts, instead of letting your thoughts master you.

# CHAPTER 6

# Reclaiming Your Autonomy

"Do not be conformed to this world, but be transformed
by the renewal of your mind, that by testing you may discern what
is the will of God, what is good and acceptable and perfect."

—Romans 12:2

IN 1966, RUBIN "Hurricane" Carter was convicted of a crime he did not commit.[26] Carter, a professional boxer best known for his in-ring personality and a vicious left hook, was thrown in prison for triple homicide. He would remain in jail for more than nineteen years. Carter's case became well-known as he fought to prove his innocence. The boxer's case made it all the way to the United States

---

26  Selwyn Raab, "Rubin (Hurricane) Carter, Boxer Found Wrongly Convicted, Dies at 76," *The New York Times*, April 22, 2014, https://www.nytimes.com/2014/04/21/sports/rubin-hurricane-carter-fearsome-boxer-dies-at-76.html.

Supreme Court where the appeal still failed. Bob Dylan wrote a song about Carter called "Hurricane" in 1976, and his story was later reenacted by Denzel Washington in a movie by a similar name.

We are not discussing Rubin "Hurricane" Carter because of his failed attempt at the Supreme Court. Indeed, the reason he is a shining example for us in our journey to end burnout is that Carter was a master of his mindset. This mastery was captured in a quote to the *New York Times* in 1977, where Carter said, "They can incarcerate my body but never my mind." Like Nelson Mandela, Carter could not control his external circumstances, but he could refuse to be a victim. They could take his professional autonomy as a boxer, but he would not let his personal autonomy be taken away. Carter's captors could control his external environment, but they could never control his internal state of being or the intention with which he lived his life.

While Carter was in prison, he made a commitment to himself that he would refuse to break, grovel, or despair. Instead, he poured his time into reading books on legal matters, philosophy, and religion. He built his legal case to prove his innocence. While he did, Carter demanded to be treated with respect. In fact, during his imprisonment, he refused to wear a prison uniform, work to reduce his prison sentence, or eat prison food. The man with a vicious left hook also told guards that if they touched him, they better be ready for a fistfight with a world-class boxer.

Instead of being a victim while in prison, Rubin "Hurricane" Carter spent every second of his time on his legal case and improving himself in any way that he could. He knew he was innocent, and, therefore, refused to be the victim. After nineteen years, his guilty verdict was finally overturned. He then went on with his life as if nothing had ever happened.

Like Carter, we may be in a terrible situation in medicine. We may be working in hospitals and clinics that continually devalue us and work to steal our professional autonomy. However, that does not mean that we have to assume the position of being a victim. Like Nelson Mandela or Rubin "Hurricane" Carter, doctors can choose to become the hero of our story despite the impossible problems caused by insurance companies, administrators, and nonclinical tasks. *While we are on the topic, don't forget about those online modules and the charting you need to complete!! Ugh.*

## THE MOST COMMON MISTAKE PHYSICIANS MAKE

From Mandela to Maya Angelou and Carter, we have seen that it is possible to simultaneously work to improve our external situations while we also refuse to be the victim *of* those situations. Unfortunately, this is not intuitive. Like the Group 2 dogs in Seligman's experiment on learned helplessness, some of us are able to escape our burnout by seeking a new situation. This could mean a new job or going part-time in medicine. For others, they transition into locum tenens work or start a side gig to create more nonclinical income. And for those who have truly had it with medicine, they leave clinical medicine altogether for things like utilization management, biotech, or Big Pharma.

However, there are many other burned-out physicians who end up being more like the Group 3 German shepherds from Seligman's experiment. These burned-out doctors have tried all the things that the Group 2 doctors have tried. Yet, they learn there is nothing they can do to change how they feel. They feel helpless, and like the Group 3 dogs, they don't fight it. They have accepted the belief that if they stay in medicine, that means being miserable. So, instead of leaving, they lie down and take it for thirty years until they can one day retire as a hollow shell of who they used to be. Trust me, I've seen it. And it isn't pretty.

What these burned-out doctors are missing—that Mandela and Carter understood—is that internal work is the key to the personal and professional autonomy we are looking to create. Remember, the idea that external circumstances do not have to control our internal feelings is not new. It has been around since the days of the ancient stoics like Epictetus over 2,000 years ago.

Yet, it wasn't until I saw this idea captured in the thought model created by Brooke Castillo, the founder of the Life Coach School, that it all clicked. When asked about the thought model I am about to show you, many of our coaching clients put it this way: "It is like seeing HD television for the first time. Once you see it, you can't *NOT* see it. It is always there." Apparently, they felt the same way about the thought model as I did about the IMAX 3D experience of *Avatar* in 2009. Once you see it, you cannot go back. Consider that your warning! Turn back now if you don't want to change your life.

## FIRST, A WORD ABOUT YOUR FEELINGS

For physicians who are struggling with burnout, they may not be able to put their finger on the cause of their problem, but they do know how they feel. This is important because, according to Douglas Lisle's motivational triad, every decision we make in our life is driven by our feelings. His triad states that every decision we make in life is driven by one of the following three motivations:

- seeking pleasure
- avoiding pain
- efficiency

For burned-out doctors, this means avoiding pain (e.g., burnout) or seeking pleasure (the things we turn to when we cannot make the pain of burnout go away). The third component of the triad is that we attempt to achieve this avoidance of pain or finding pleasure as efficiently as we can. This is the reason that some doctors turn to alcohol when they aren't willing to feel the stress caused by their situation. Alcohol—like many emotional buffers—is highly efficient in helping us escape feelings that we are not willing to feel. Like the profit-focused model discussed in this book, however, buffers like alcohol are a short-term fix with grave long-term consequences.

The motivational triad explains why so many doctors, who work on average sixty hours per week, will spend *more* time building nonclinical streams of income, even when they are overworked and stressed out. Many doctors are looking for a way to work for themselves, instead of working for a system that abuses them. As we have discussed at length, autonomy is supremely important to living a life of self-determination. Working for yourself is a means of escape. As *Shark Tank's* Lori Greiner put it in a *Business Insider* interview, "I have a quote that I always say, that I love, which is, 'Entrepreneurs are the only people who will work eighty hours a week to avoid working forty hours a week'...And it is true, because we like to be our own bosses."[27]

Each decision we make is driven by our desire to seek pleasure, avoid pain, and to do either of these things as efficiently as possible. This line of logic only makes sense, however, if we view our feelings as automatic. In Kahneman and Tversky's words, are our feelings all System 2 feelings? Or do we have intentional control over them? In other words, do our feelings control us, or do we control our feelings?

## THE THOUGHT MODEL

Many of us go through life beholden to the events that happen around us. Things that are completely out of our control seem to

---

27  Libby Kane, "'Shark Tank' Investor: 'Entrepreneurs are the only people who will work 80 hours a week to avoid working 40 hours a week," *Business Insider*, July 13, 2016, https://www.businessinsider.com/lori-greiner-shark-tank-entrepreneurs-2016-7.

dictate our thoughts, feelings, and actions. This has a way of sneaking into our everyday language, too. We talk about how angry our spouse makes us. Or how overwhelmed we feel when our employer adds one more requirement to our already full plate. *What?!? You still haven't finished all of your online modules yet?* Maybe you have kids and you get easily annoyed when your children don't listen, start bickering, or start kicking the back of your seat when you drive.

Whatever the situation, this sort of thinking implies one fatally flawed concept—that our circumstances determine our thoughts, feelings, actions, and results. This is the problem. When we feel that life is happening *to* us and not *for* us, it is easy to feel like the victim of a bad situation. When we let our external situations in life determine how we feel, we feel powerless. This is the basis for the learned helplessness and the victim mentality that we have discussed at length in this book. It is as if we have no control over how we feel. Is that really what we want? Enter here Brooke Castillo's thought model.

Let's explore the thought model through an example. Let's say that you are driving in the right lane on the interstate when the car next to you speeds up and cuts you off for no apparent reason. Immediately, you feel your anger start to boil over. It starts with a clenched jaw and a tight grip on the steering wheel. After a few choice words, it may involve trying to get back at the scoundrel in front of you. They clearly have no respect for your life or your safety. You will show this guy!

When you get to work, you are still upset about the incident. *"You would not believe this guy on the interstate today. He cut me off for no reason. What an idiot. I am so mad!"*

Let's break down this common, everyday life event—and the language we use surrounding it. In the example above, you think that the person driving the car who cut you off made you angry. As Jon Acuff would encourage us to ask, "Is that really true?" Said differently, is it factual?

Here is what actually happened in objective terms: While driving in the right lane, a car passed you on the left. It then shifted lanes within ten feet of your front bumper. This was the circumstance, or the verifiable facts that two lawyers would agree on in a court of law. It is measurable and objective. After this event, you had a chance to decide whether that action constituted being "cut off." *Is it five feet, ten feet, or twenty feet in front of your bumper that counts as being cut off? What about fifty feet?*

Then, a thought entered your mind. Maybe you thought, *That person clearly doesn't care about my safety.* Or perhaps, *Didn't that guy see me? He doesn't respect me or my space.* It could also have been as simple as *What a jerk!*

That thought then produced a feeling—anger in this situation. As your jaw started to clench and your hands tightened around the steering wheel, your anger then led you to take action. You shifted into the left lane, punched the gas pedal to the floorboard, and gave the person in the lane next to you the one-finger salute. *Take that!*

The end result is that you endangered your own safety, which I'll remind you is why you were mad in the first place when the person in the other lane did the same. You were then fully engaged in a road-rage battle. In addition to that, long after the event, the person who cut you off was still controlling how you felt when you got to work. How's that working out for you?

What I just walked you through is called the thought model. It is one of the tools we use in coaching our physician clients. It follows an acronym: CTFAR.[28] Let's break it down, and then we can fill in the model for our story above.

---

28  This is the Thought Model taught by The Life Coach School. The Life Coach School is also where I spent six months earning my coaching certification. For more information, visit https://thelifecoachschool.com/.

| CTFAR THOUGHT MODEL | |
|---|---|
| C = Circumstances | Undeniable, verifiable facts. |
| T = Thought | What you think about a circumstance. |
| F = Feeling | The feeling produced by the thought. |
| A = Action | The action (or inaction) that results from your feeling. |
| R = Result | The outcome of the action. |

So, looking at our example above, this is what it would look like:

| CTFAR THOUGHT MODEL | |
|---|---|
| Circumstance | A car shifted lanes in front of your car within ten feet of your front bumper. |
| Thought | "This idiot doesn't respect me or my safety!" |
| Feeling | Anger |
| Action | You shifted lanes, sped ahead, flipped off the other driver, and cut him off in return. |
| Result | You endanger your safety. |

Now, I'd be willing to wager that when you started your day, you didn't think, *You know what I want to do today? I want to get angry on the road and get into a dangerous high-speed battle with a random person on the interstate!* No? You mean that wasn't what you were hoping for when you rolled out of bed?

The thought model can be a tough pill for people to swallow at first. This is because once we see it, we realize what Mandela, Carter, and the ancient stoics like Epictetus all understood. It is not our external circumstances that cause our feelings. It is our *thought* about the circumstances that does.

In the road rage example, it was not the person cutting you off that made you mad. It was your thought about it that led to the anger.

In between your external circumstance and your action, there was an opportunity to dictate your internal dialogue. Like Epictetus said 2,000 years ago, the chief task in life is to figure out which things are external to us that we cannot control and which are the internal choices we can control—like our thoughts, feelings, and actions.

In the thought model above, the circumstance is objective. As I have said countless times in life to my kids, "It is what it is." The car passed you on your left and shifted lanes in front of you within ten feet of your front bumper. You cannot change that. It is a verifiable fact that any two people could measure and agree upon. However, that circumstance does not, in and of itself, dictate your feelings and actions. Those, my friend, are dictated by your thoughts. I don't want to gloss over this point, because it is important, and it can either serve as a great source of frustration or it can allow you to reclaim your personal and professional autonomy.

Whenever I say "It is what it is" in my household, my wife Kristen always follows that comment up with "but it will be what you make it." There is a lot of wisdom in that. So, let's go back to our interstate example and see if it is what it is or if it will be what we make it. When that car shifted lanes within ten feet of your front bumper, that part remains a fact. It is what it is. However, there is an infinite number of thoughts we could have chosen that would have created very different feelings, actions, and results. For example, we could have thought, *Maybe that guy's wife is in labor and he is in a hurry to make it to the hospital.* Or perhaps, *He is probably running late...I've totally been there*, or maybe the simplest of all explanations, *I bet he didn't realize how close he was to me when he shifted lanes. Maybe he didn't see me.*

All of these thoughts produce a very different kind of feeling, don't they? It will be what we make it, right? Some thoughts produce compassion and empathy like, *Hey, I've been late before.* Other thoughts produce understanding: *Maybe he just didn't see me.* One thing is clear, however. It is your thoughts that determine your feelings. Not your external circumstances.

You might feel empathy for the driver's pregnant wife having their first child. You may feel compassion as he is in a rush to work because the alarm didn't go off. Maybe you have been in some of the same situations. When you experience compassion or empathy instead of anger, it is not because the circumstance changed. It is because your thoughts about the circumstance changed.

Different thoughts, even in the same situation, produce different feelings. When we replace anger with empathy or compassion, we are unlikely to speed up and cut the guy off in return. We are even less likely to engage in a high-speed road-rage battle. In fact, we will probably keep cruising along while singing our favorite new song at the top of our lungs or listening to our favorite book or podcast. Just like we were before the car shifted in front of us. We don't have to be the victim of our circumstances. Instead, we can be the hero just like Nelson Mandela, Maya Angelou, or Rubin "Hurricane" Carter.

The point is this: When we continue to think that it is our circumstances, not our thoughts, that determine our feelings, then we continually hand over the keys to our feelings to people and events we cannot control. The importance of this point cannot be overstated. If we want to reclaim our personal and professional autonomy even when our healthcare organizations continue to place their focus on profit over people, this is the first step in doing that.

## FROM VICTIM TO VICTOR

What attracted me to anesthesiology was that it requires quick action while figuring out the ultimate problem. While many medical specialties tend to operate in a "think first, then act" style of practice, anesthesia is often the opposite. Anesthesiologists are often required to act first (e.g., bolus some phenylephrine) while we simultaneously try to figure out the cause of the problem (e.g., hypotension). However, if we stop at treating the symptom, and fail to diagnose the problem, this is not practicing medicine. We all recognize that treating symptoms instead of the disease is rarely helpful in terms of the big picture.

Yet, this is exactly what most physicians do when it comes to their burnout. They blame their lack of autonomy, belonging, and perceived competence on their external circumstances (which they cannot control) instead of focusing on the real problem at hand (their internal thoughts, perspectives, and paradigms about their external circumstances). When Rubin "Hurricane" Carter and Nelson Mandela recognized that they were in prison, we can all agree that it was a circumstantial fact. It was something that happened to them externally that two lawyers, even if on opposing sides, would agree on in a court of law. Yet, they realized that the biggest problem was not their imprisonment but how they *viewed* their imprisonment.

In coaching, this idea of making the diagnosis in order to provide the proper solution is called "causal" coaching. In causal coaching, time is spent separating the facts (circumstances) from the story (our thoughts about those circumstances). This kind of coaching focuses on the thought that is causing our problems. By the way, the alternative to causal coaching is when a coach simply tells you what actions to take, and I don't recommend it. Advice-based coaching is a short-term fix, not a long-term solution. The long-term solution involves finding the cause of our feelings, actions, and results—our thoughts.

Think about it. Can you imagine how different South Africa would be if Nelson Mandela spent all of his time complaining about his situation and perseverating on how unjust it was? He would have been consumed by the bitterness Maya Angelou warned us against. What if Mandela never focused on his anti-apartheid efforts that attached him to his deeper purpose? This could only be done from a position of strength, not from labeling himself as a victim.

## SAL'S STORY

Once, I was coaching a primary care physician during a group coaching call. In order to protect the innocent, let's call this client Sal. Sal's partner was on vacation, and so he was covering for this other doc while they were away. During this time, a patient of the other doctor's called to have their opioid prescription increased. The office policy at the time was that, while away, partners would not make changes to opioid regimens for long-term chronic pain patients. So, when the patient asked to increase their opioid prescription, Sal told the patient that based on policy, they would be unable to. The patient then asked for a second opinion, and one of Sal's colleagues agreed that no increase was warranted or reasonable at that time. Getting yet a third opinion from another colleague, the patient eventually found a physician in the group who agreed to increase their dose.

Sal was upset and felt that this colleague was enabling bad patient behavior. Many of the other clients on the group call felt the same way and said so in the chat section. Remember, my job as a coach is to be a curious skeptic about Sal's story. Sal had already believed this narrative that the third partner was enabling the patient, and it was making Sal angry. So, I asked if there was any way he could give this third colleague the benefit of the doubt. Was there any way Sal could view this situation more charitably? When looking for alternative explanations for why a perfectly reasonable, intelligent partner that Sal trusted might do something like this, they realized that the third partner may have received different information. Sal also thought it was possible that the doc who increased the opioid script may have talked to the primary doctor who was on vacation. Maybe they got permission to increase the prescription? The more Sal thought about it, the more he realized that there were a number of reasons his partner could have increased the script.

Ultimately, Sal realized that by thinking his partner was enabling bad patient behavior, he was handing the keys to his feelings over to someone else to determine how he felt. Sal didn't want this. Like the person shifting lanes in front of you on the interstate, Sal could choose to provide the benefit of the doubt or to find out what actually happened and address it with that partner. What the partner did wasn't the cause of the anger that Sal felt. The cause of Sal's anger was filling in the gaps of this situation with his narrative about enabling bad patient behavior.

Unfortunately, this is what human minds are wired to do. When given information, our minds will fill in any gaps we find, often with the worst possible narrative. In Sal's situation, the gap in the information he had was filled in with a narrative about his partner enabling bad patient behavior. This put his professional autonomy (not being overridden by a partner) and his sense of belonging (now that he was at odds with the partner) in jeopardy. Sal could let this serve as one of the thousands of paper cuts that would lead to burnout, or he could choose to fix the cause—his thoughts about the situation.

This habit our brain has for filling in gaps is not new. It has always been there. You may remember a viral email that made its way around the internet in 2003 that proved this point. In the email was a paragraph that consisted of words where the letters were scrambled. Yet, despite very few of the words being spelled correctly, people could read it with ease. This neologism is called typoglycemia, which is the ability humans have to read words and paragraphs with jumbled-up letters without any problem. As long as the words are short, first letters remain the same, and function words like "a" and "the" remain correct, our minds are wired to recognize patterns. My point is that when we have limited information, our brains are very good at filling in the gaps. This is how we make sense of stories when we don't have all of the information.

For those who are interested, here is an example of typoglycemia from that viral email in 2003:

Aoccdrnig to a rscheearch at Cmabrigde Uinervtisy, it deosn't mttaer in waht oredr the ltteers in a wrod are, the olny iprmoetnt tihng is taht the frist and lsat ltteer be at the rghit pclae. The rset can be a toatl mses and you can sitll raed it wouthit porbelm. Tihs is bcuseae the huamn mnid deos not raed ervey lteter by istlef, but the wrod as a wlohe.[29]

Unfortunately, most of the time, these thoughts that fill in the gaps are overwhelmingly negative. None of us are immune to this, and in fact, that is exactly what I did when I wasn't selected for one of the Assistant Program Director positions. It took a friend (and multiple coaching sessions) to help me see that the terrible reasons my mind was coming up with for why I wasn't chosen were full of fictional thoughts and very few facts. I was upset not because I didn't get chosen but because my brain was filling in the few facts I had with the worst imaginable story.

When we find ourselves in this trap, we can choose a different thought, soundtrack, or story. As a way of practical application for when you feel stuck in a negative thought pattern, here are some helpful questions you might ask to help you flip your focus:

- How is this happening *for* me, instead of *to* me?
- Is this really true?
- Do I want to believe this?
- Is there any possible good that is coming out of this event?
- Of all the thoughts in the world that I can choose to think about this situation, why am I choosing this one?

---

29  Dictionary.com, s.v. "If Yuo're Albe To Raed Tihs, You Might Have Typoglycemia," January 21, 2021, https://www.dictionary.com/e/typoglycemia/.

While hindsight is 20/20, we often don't have the perspective we need in real time. Regardless of how you flip your perspective or paradigm about the situation, the truth remains. It is our thoughts that control our feelings, not our circumstances. And this fundamental understanding has the power to give you personal and professional autonomy. However, in order to do this, you will need to learn about the difference between unintentional and intentional thoughts.

# CHAPTER 7

# From System 2 to System 1

"I found that when you start thinking and saying what you really want then your mind automatically shifts and pulls you in that direction. And sometimes it can be that simple, just a little twist in vocabulary that illustrates your attitude and philosophy."
—Jim Rohn

IN THE 1980S, a study was performed that gave lung cancer patients two choices. They could either pursue surgery or they could choose radiation based on the following information. The study was broken up into two groups. In the first group, information was framed positively. This is what they were told:

> **Surgery:** Of 100 people having surgery, ninety live through the postoperative period, sixty-eight are alive at the end of the first year, and thirty-four are alive at the end of five years.

Radiation Therapy: Of 100 people having radiation
therapy, all live through the treatment, seventy-seven are
alive at the end of one year, and twenty-two are alive at the
end of five years.

Note that this is framed in terms of the percentage of patients
who would survive. If patients pursued surgery, they could expect
to survive 90% of the time after one year and 34% could expect to be
alive at five years. In radiation therapy, 77% are alive after one year,
but only 22% are alive at five years. When presented using survival
rates, a mere 18% of participants in the study chose radiation even
though it had a 12% lower five-year survival rate.

In the second group, a negative frame was used where information was given in terms of mortality, instead of with a positive survival frame. This is what they were told:

Surgery: Of 100 people having surgery, ten die during surgery or the postoperative period, thirty-two die by the end
of the first year, and sixty-six die by the end of five years.

Radiation Therapy: Of 100 people having radiation
therapy, none die during treatment, twenty-three die by
the end of one year, and seventy-eight die by the end of
five years.

It is important to note that the statistics given in the negative
frame are the same as in the first half of the experiment. They are
simply framed in terms of mortality instead of survival. When
framed negatively, 10% of patients die immediately after surgery
while none die after radiation. At one year, 32% of patients die
after surgery compared to 23% who received radiation. And at five
years, mortality is 12% higher in the radiation group. When framed
through a mortality lens, the number of patients who chose radia-

tion skyrocketed from 18% to 44% because patients were faced with a 10% chance of mortality immediately following surgery. Said differently, patients were more than twice as likely to choose radiation, despite a lower five-year rate of survival, when the same mortality statistics were framed negatively.

There are a couple of take-home messages here. First, be careful how you speak to patients when obtaining consent for procedures as it turns out how you frame your words has an impact on their decision. When you tell someone they have a 90% chance of survival, they are much more likely to consent for a procedure than if you tell them they have a 10% chance of death. You likely already knew that, though.

The second take-home point is that words—and the focus these words produce—are powerful. The study mentioned above[30] was conducted by Daniel Kahneman and Amos Tversky, the two Israeli psychologists we introduced previously who spent their life's work studying decision-making and coined the System 1 and System 2 decision-making processes. Their findings are fascinating. Kahneman would eventually win the Nobel Prize for their work. Tversky would have received the same, but he unfortunately died from metastatic melanoma before the award was given.

In *Thinking, Fast and Slow*, Kahneman describes much of the work that he and Tversky published during their time working together. We discussed earlier that Kahneman describes the two systems we use to make decisions as System 1 and System 2 thinking.

Recall that System 1 is described as fast, automatic, and emotional. System 1 is the system we use when someone says, "Think

30   Amos Tversky and Daniel Kahneman, "Rational Choice and the Framing of Decisions," *The Journal of Business* 59, no. 4, part 2: The Behavioral Foundations of Economic Theory, (October, 1986): S251–S278, https://www.jstor.org/stable/2352759?seq=1.

fast!" and throws a ball our way and we somehow catch it. System 1 is also the system you were using to drive your car on the interstate before that guy cut you off in the previous chapter. It is instinctive. Examples we discussed earlier that Kahneman gives to show this sort of thinking also include the following:

- Solve 2 + 2 = ?
- Finish the phrase, "War and..."

Remember that if you answered that 2 + 2 = 4 or you said "War and Peace," then you were using System 1. This is automatic work that requires very little effort on our part. It happens without a second thought and requires little attention or energy. On the other hand, System 2 is slow, methodical, and logical. It is the system we use to make complicated executive decisions. Examples in the same realm shown above that would employ the use of System 2 include:

- Solving 17 × 24
- Parallel parking in a tight space
- Counting the number of "As" in the following paragraph

All of these examples require you to focus intently on your work. These are the situations that make it difficult to chew bubble gum and walk. It requires attention to detail and focus to get it right. Fortunately, we can switch back and forth between System 1 and System 2 when the need arises. When it comes to thought work, it requires us to "unlearn" the current System 1 thinking that leads to our perspectives, paradigms, and stories that our thoughts are unintentionally producing right now. And to "relearn" a new System 2 style of thinking that is intentional. It will be slow and methodical at first but—if practiced—will transition into automatic System 1 thinking.

*By the way, there are thirty-eight "As" in the previous paragraph;*

*17 × 24 = 408; and, no, I cannot help you parallel park into that tight parking spot.*

## UNINTENTIONAL TO INTENTIONAL THOUGHT MODELS

James Clear, the author of *Atomic Habits*, defines a habit this way, "A habit is a routine or behavior that is performed regularly and, in many cases, automatically."

When working with physician clients, our goal is to find their unintentional thought models that occur via System 1 thinking and result in their automatic habits, feelings, actions, and results. Then, if they want, we help them unlearn this unhelpful narrative so that they can replace it with an intentional System 2 thought that produces the feelings, actions, and results that they want. This is what we call transitioning from an unintentional thought model to an intentional thought model.

For example, let's say you find yourself drinking two or three beers every night when you get home because there is currently a pandemic and you have three young kids in virtual learning at home. *Why are you looking at me? I'm not stressed out! You're stressed out!* In this environment, drinking might not feel like a choice. It is something we automatically do when the stress rises. It happens *to* us and seems completely involuntary. In other words, it is an automatic habit.

This habit of daily drinking occurs automatically via System 1. It is possible that we have never taken a moment to stop and think about why we are having the drinks every night in the first place. If unexamined, we might not consider that the cause of our drinking is stress. And that the feeling of stress came from a very automatic and unintentional thought. If we never do the thought work to figure out the root cause that is driving the stress, we can't make the right diagnosis to solve the problem. Remember, our thoughts are a choice. What if we change our thoughts?

What if we decide very intentionally, *I am not going to drink any alcoholic beverages unless I decide twenty-four hours in advance what I am going to drink, how much I'll drink, and why.*

When we decide *a priori* that we will not let our circumstances and emotions dictate our actions, and that instead we are going to be intentional about our drinking, it can change our actions. This allows us to stop the automatic feedback loop of stress → urge → response. This system, which often runs on autopilot, makes us feel like we have no control over whether we drink or not. It can be reversed.

Instead, we'll drink when we are completely in control of our decision-making (i.e., before we have the first drink) and well before our circumstances ever happen. This intentional System 2 thought process allows us to remain in control and is followed by actions and results that we would be proud to show our family. This can be a very powerful cycle of intrinsic motivation as our competence to drink intentionally increases. Will we always get it right? Probably not. But each time we do, it is a vote for the kind of person we are working to become. The goal is to put more votes in the direction we are heading than we do in the opposite direction.

While just an example, this process of unlearning System 1 thoughts and relearning System 2 thought patterns can help burned-out doctors. In the same way we learned how to drive a car or learned how to perform medical procedures, we can take what used to be a slow and methodical process and learn how to make it an automatic habit. In order to do this when it comes to burnout, we must first discover the System 1 focus that is driving our feelings and actions. Only then can our System 1 thought be unlearned and then replaced with an intentional System 2 thought process. The cool part is that once the original thought is unlearned and replaced with a System 2 thought, we can work to practice that System 2 thought until it becomes automatic and continually produces the feelings, actions, and results we desire.

In fact, this process is one and the same with the now well-described practice of positive affirmations. Admittedly, when I first heard about positive affirmations, I thought it was ridiculous, but after being coached myself and coaching other burned-out doctors, I've realized what the science has already shown to be true. When we replace unhelpful thoughts with ones that produce the results we want in our life, it is liberating.

In fact, functional MRI studies have shown that when people practice replacing their unhelpful thoughts with intentionally positive affirmations, the dopaminergic reward system lights up. Positive self-talk has also been shown to decrease stress, increase how much people exercise, improve eating habits, and even help people achieve more academically. You can think of positive affirmations as brain hacks for accomplishing our goals. It may sound woo-woo to you, like it used to for me, but it works. And I am all about the stuff that works.

As an example, here are some of the positive affirmations (or "zingers" as some of my clients like to call them) I use that produce positive results in my life and help me work toward becoming a more self-determined husband, father, and physician each day:

- When I say "no" to one thing, I am saying "Hell Yes" to what matters most.
- Pivot, don't panic. (When life throws you a curveball.)
- It is about getting it right, not being right. (Stolen in full transparency from Brené Brown...seriously, go and read her books already!)
- Self-care is not selfish.
- This is happening *for* me, not *to* me.
- The obstacle isn't *in* the way, it is *the* way to success.
- Start before you're ready. Start by starting. Start now. (*Physician Philosopher* podcast fans will recognize this one.)
- You cannot know success without knowing failure.

Finding the unintentional thoughts that are running amok in our life and replacing them with intentionally focused perspectives, thoughts, and affirmations that will serve us is exactly what the doctor ordered. If you think this all sounds ridiculous, I only ask you to try it. Say some positive affirmations in front of the mirror each day. Join a coaching program that can help you focus (or find) the narrative that is most helpful for you in your current situation.

Is it easy work weeding out the destructive thoughts and replacing them with intentional thoughts that serve us? No. But most things in life that are worth the outcome require some amount of hard work. Thought work is more a marathon than a sprint. It is an iterative process that becomes easier and easier with practice. While we won't win every battle, with each decision we make, we are voting for the kind of person we are working to become. With hard work, we can send more votes in the direction of becoming a self-determined physician than toward the burned-out narrative we have carried for so long.

This does beg the question, what if we have done the thought work and we think our circumstance still needs to change? Aren't there times where replacing the thought isn't enough? That's what we will talk about next.

# PART 4

# POWERFUL PARADIGMS

I PREVIOUSLY MENTIONED Jon Acuff's book *Soundtracks: The Surprising Solution to Overthinking*. In it, Acuff lays out the argument that the cause of overthinking is a broken soundtrack, or repetitive thought patterns that prevent us from moving on. These broken soundtracks, however, do not mean that our *brain* is broken. When we get stuck in a repetitive yet unhelpful thought pattern, our brain is doing what it is supposed to do.

See, our brain has two principal jobs. Our brain's first job is to act like a machine, or to perform the process of thinking. As Acuff's subtitle points out, this is something our brain has the propensity to turn into overthinking. Our brain doesn't care what it is thinking; it just cares that it *is* thinking. It is a machine. A really impressive machine, but a machine nonetheless. However, if our brain is left to its own devices, it will produce whatever narrative happens to come into focus.

Our brain's second job is to fulfill the mission set out by Lisle's motivational triad: to seek pleasure, avoid pain, and to do either of these tasks as efficiently as possible. Specifically, our brain's second function is to protect us from harm. While this protective function may have been useful to our ancestors when we were hunters and gatherers, it doesn't always prove helpful in modern times. Our ancestors needed constant vigilance against lions and tigers and bears (*oh my!*). *We* often do not. Yet, our brain still has a function to fill, and when no danger is present, it will work to convince us that isn't the case. This is when we start to overthink.

Acuff's solution for this is to replace our broken soundtracks with soundtracks that resonate with who we are, who we want to become, and what we are trying to accomplish in life. You'll note the similarity here with what we have discussed in this book from the world of coaching. Coaching helps clients identify the unintentional thoughts that are harming them and encourages them to consider replacing these thoughts with intentional thoughts that will serve them instead. Stephen Covey, the author of *The 7 Habits of Highly Effective People*, referred to this as changing paradigms or perspectives. Tversky and Kahneman called this the work of transitioning from System 1 to System 2 thinking.

Whether we are following the teachings of Acuff, Covey, or Castillo, the theme remains. We all have soundtracks, paradigms, and thoughts that can lead us astray. That's why in the final part of this book, we will discuss some of the most common unintentional models that plague the physician community. Then, we will discuss some of the tools we use to help our physician clients replace these broken paradigms with new ones that will serve them. It is through these powerful paradigms that we can work toward becoming self-determined physicians, even if our healthcare organizations refuse to change.

Everything we discuss here will be aimed at helping you work toward mastering the ABCs of becoming more self-determined, which I have adapted from the original work of Edward Deci and Richard Ryan. Each chapter, then, will help you either reclaim your autonomy, discover a deeper sense of belonging, or improve your real or perceived competence. Since I believe in the saying "Brevity is the soul of wit," I have aimed to include some of the higher-yield nuggets we often teach our clients, but this is not an exhaustive list. Let's dive into some of the most common tools we use to help physicians create a life they love.

# CHAPTER 8

# The Best Teacher

"Everything negative—pressure, challenges—
is all an opportunity for me to rise."
—Kobe Bryant

MY PARENTS MADE one thing clear when my sisters and I became old enough to drive. If we got a ticket, they would take away our car (*let's be real; it was their car*). So, when my sister Kristin got her first speeding ticket, it made for an interesting situation. Kristin had a job working as a waitress. She also had a social life as a junior in high school. She didn't want to lose her car. Naturally, this was a very stressful situation for Kristin. *For those paying attention, yes, my sister's name is the same as my wife's. Technically, they are homophones as they are spelled differently. When my grandfather was alive, he used to call my wife Kristen "E-N" and my sister Kristin "I-N" to distinguish the two.*

With the new ticket, Kristin (or "I-N") was appropriately worried. Knowing she had time before the ticket had to be paid, she picked up some extra shifts at her job while she hid the ticket from our parents. Then, she signed up for a class that would remove the points from her license. After she had accumulated enough money, she sat down to write a letter to our parents. In the letter, she told them that she had made a mistake but that she had also accepted the responsibility. She further explained that she had worked some extra shifts to earn enough money to pay for the ticket and had signed up for a class with the local DMV offered by the state of Florida to remove the points she would receive. This way, her insurance premium would not increase. After writing the letter, she placed it into an envelope along with the money required to pay for the ticket. Then, Kristin taped the envelope to our parents' bedroom door.

When Mom and Dad woke up the next day, they had zero issue with what Kristin had done. Because of how Kristin handled what would have otherwise been a fairly negative experience, our parents required no consequence. Through this challenge, Kristin learned about responsibility and accountability. These skills would serve her well as she found success in her career while becoming a badass single mom a few years later in life. In other words, she refused to let a potentially negative experience dictate her outcome. Instead, she used her autonomy and viewed her speeding ticket as an opportunity to learn.

Kristin did not solve her problem despite the stress caused by her situation. No, she solved the problem *because* of the stress she felt. In other words, despite the anxiety associated with her situation, she decided to pivot instead of panicking. She turned her negative experience into a positive result. This concept that negative feelings can actually produce positive results is something we focus on when coaching our physician clients.

For example, we commonly take our clients through an exercise to help them process the negative feelings many physicians experience. This could be feelings that arise from burnout or possible career transitions. It could also be the stress caused by a difficult situation at home or at work. Like Kristin with her speeding ticket, we help a lot of doctors turn negative feelings into positive results.

In order to avoid poisoning the well, let's go through an exercise.

What I want you to do is to answer the following questions. You can write them down (or say them out loud if you are driving a car while listening to the audio version of this book). In order to do this, pause after each question and determine your answers before proceeding to the next.

The first question is this: on a daily or weekly basis, what three feelings or emotions do you most commonly feel? Do you most often feel anger, angst, anxiety, stress, and overwhelm? Or is it joy, contentment, happiness, and peace? Out of the multitude of possible emotions or feelings you could experience each day, what are the top three? What comes to mind? Reflect on this for a moment, then write these three feelings or emotions down (or hit pause and say them aloud):

1.

2.

3.

The second question is slightly different. What three feelings would you *like to* feel most commonly on a daily or weekly basis? Notice that this is what you want, not what you actually feel. Take a moment to pause, and then write down (or say aloud) the top three feelings that you would like to experience on a daily or weekly basis:

1.

2.

3.

After you have your two lists, look at them closely. If you are like the hundreds of doctors we have coached, I bet you'll see a pattern. In the first exercise regarding the top three feelings you actually feel on a daily or weekly basis, I bet at least two of the three are negative. You may have listed things like anxiety, overwhelm, stress, fear, depression, or frustration. For some physicians, all three are negative. When you look at your list, how does it hold up? Were two of the three feelings negative? Was at least one of them negative?

With the second question regarding the three feelings you *want* to feel most commonly, I am willing to bet that all three were positive. Most often, it will be things like fulfillment, satisfaction, joy, happiness, contentment, hope, or love. When you note the juxtaposition of the first and second lists, it's fascinating, isn't it? How is it that what we most commonly experience is, on average, mostly negative and what we want to feel each day is universally positive? Is that just the way life is? Do we really only want to feel positive emotions?

## NEGATIVE FEELINGS, POSITIVE RESULTS

Earlier in this book we introduced the concept of the motivational triad. As a reminder, this is the theory that states that our decisions in life are driven by our motivation to seek pleasure, avoid pain, and accomplish either of these tasks as efficiently as possible. This triad implies a truth that you just experienced—we all want to feel positive feelings and avoid negative feelings 100% of the time. If left to our own devices, every decision we make would follow this pattern.

However, this doesn't really hold up. Wanting all positive and no negative feelings is a bit like communism. Good in theory, but terrible in practice. Communism supports the notion that everyone should be taken care of regardless of their social class, occupation, productivity, or station in life. Wouldn't we all agree that sounds great? Yet, communism is terrible in reality. It turns out that no one works hard when we all get the same reward regardless of how hard we work. The narrative that we want to avoid negative feelings 100% of the time is similarly good in theory, but terrible in reality. While we may tell ourselves we don't like negative feelings, the truth is that we actually *want* to experience negative feelings.

I was born and raised in the South. My sisters and I were raised to say "Yes, ma'am" and "No, ma'am" instead of "Yes" or "No." If we didn't hear what Mom said, the appropriate thing to say wasn't

"What did you say?" It was to say, "Ma'am?" Call me old-fashioned, but I appreciate some of the lessons that those traditions taught me. Things like respect, selflessness, and a family-first approach to life.

It should come as no surprise then that when I decided I was going to propose to Kristen (E-N), I felt that the traditional course of action was to ask her mom and dad for their blessing. So, like the band Magic's famous song "Rude," I put on my best suit, got in my car, and raced down to South Carolina.

Upon arriving, as the lyrics go, my heart was in my hand. I was extremely nervous about the whole thing. Kristen's parents can be challenging to read. They keep a lot of their feelings close to the vest. So, believe it or not, I had no idea what they would say. Despite my nerves (or maybe because of them, we will come to find out), I found the courage to ask for permission to marry their daughter. And unlike Magic, I didn't have to ask why they had to be so rude. Fortunately, my future mother- and father-in-law said yes, but not before I ended up choking on a piece of steak, a story that still lives in family folklore. To this day, my family loves giving me a hard time for literally "choking" while I was asking to marry Kristen.

What you'll notice here is that in order to get to what I wanted most in my life, which was to marry the person who remains my much better half to this day, I had to get through or at least coexist with an otherwise unwanted emotion, being nervous. On the other side of that feeling was something I wanted much more—to feel like I belonged with my new family when they gave me their blessing to propose to Kristen. In fact, this is how much of life goes, isn't it? In order to experience the success, goals, and accomplishments that we want, we often have to work through negative feelings.

For example, as an author and podcaster, I frequently receive requests for public speaking at various conferences and grand rounds. Departments and institutions also ask me to help them with their culture. All of this involves quite a bit of public speaking. Yet, when I first started speaking publicly in college, I hated it. It was nerve-racking. This was a skill I could cultivate and hone, and I hoped that with time, the anxiety associated with public speaking would become easier. To this day, I still get nervous prior to public-speaking events. Yet, I've learned that the nervousness I have prior to big moments in life is not something to be avoided. In fact, it is usually a sign that I am about to take part in something worthwhile.

These are two examples of how a "negative" feeling can actually lead to positive results. I am sure that you can think of many more examples from your own life. What was it like when you proposed to your partner? Were you nervous? What about when you had your first kid? Did you stand over their bed at night watching them breathe only to realize that you have never been more terrified, while simultaneously filled with joy, in your whole life? Do you remember how it felt when you first became a resident and had to make medical decisions? Or the first time you operated on a patient or made a diagnosis on a tough case as an attending physician? On the other side of life's nerve-racking experiences is the stuff that matters most to us. These negative feelings are often guideposts that indicate we are on the right track. We don't want to avoid them. Instead, we need to embrace them.

Ramit Sethi, an entrepreneur and author of the book *I Will Teach You to Be Rich*, noticed this same phenomenon, which is why he created a "failure file." Sethi realized that most of his biggest successes were often preceded by some pretty epic failures. So, instead of avoiding these failures, Sethi created a failure file on his computer with a goal of creating a certain number of epic fails each month that he could place into this file. Was Sethi crazy?

Well, no. Sethi simply realized that, like the nervous energy many of us have before big moments in our life, failure was a sign that he was pushing his business to the edge. He was trying new and innovative ideas. Some of these irons in the fire would catch, others would not. Yet, Sethi realized that in order to find the good ideas, failure was a necessary part of the work. That's why each month he set a goal for the number of epic fails he was trying to achieve. And with each fail, he would celebrate the fact that he had tried something new.

There is one particular exception worth mentioning. Not all negative feelings lead to positive results. Sometimes they lead to never-ending cycles that fuel the flame of perseveration. These are called indulgent feelings or emotions, which can be defined as negative feelings that do not lead to positive results. Indulgent emotions include overwhelm, worry, doubt, and shame. When these feelings arise, the goal isn't to work through them knowing that what we want is waiting on the other side. Instead, the work is to figure out what unintentional thought is driving these indulgent emotions and then to get rid of it. In other words, indulgent emotions happen when we have broken stories, perspectives, paradigms, or soundtracks. Playing them on repeat isn't helpful.

## WHAT NEGATIVE FEELINGS ARE YOU AVOIDING?

Anesthesiology is sometimes described as a job that is 99% boredom and 1% terror. When I wrote my personal statement for residency, I referred to this and linked it back to my time as a college goalkeeper on my Division-II soccer team at Erskine College. I made the point in my personal statement that this widely held story about terror and boredom in anesthesia is only true to those who aren't actually anesthesiologists. Why? Because what makes an anesthesiologist great isn't handling the 1% of terror. While good anesthesiologists (and goalkeepers) can save anything, a great anesthesiologist is able to prevent the save from ever being necessary. That's the 99% non-anesthesiologists don't see, and in anesthesiology, it is what separates the wheat from the chaff.

However hard we may try, though, terror still happens. When it does, the best anesthesiologists remain cool, calm, and collected. And for good reason. Can you imagine an anesthesiologist who couldn't tolerate the moments of sheer terror in the operating room? What if they said, "Nope, I am not willing to deal with this stressful situation right now in order to save that patient's life!" Would you want to work with that anesthesiologist or have them save your life? I know I wouldn't.

Instead, great anesthesiologists are like the Marines in their commercial that says, "There are a few who move toward the sounds of chaos, waiting to respond at a moment's notice." In a strange way, anesthesiologists have to enjoy moving toward stressful situations, knowing that on the other side of that stress is the opportunity to help a patient in their greatest moment of need.

If working through negative feelings produces the positive results we want, why then does our brain tell us to run in the other direction in times of great stress? The answer is that our brain is a machine, and its main job is to protect us from harm. Sometimes this is good, like when we touch a hot stove, we then remember to never do that again. Other times, our brains' desire to protect us proves less helpful. For example, when we were toddlers learning how to walk, stopping at our first sign of failure would not have produced the walking result we wanted. If we stopped trying the first time we fell over because we got hurt, we might still be crawling to this day. Or the first time we kissed someone, gave a public speech, performed an operation, ran a clinic, asked for a promotion, or had to deal with the stress of an upcoming deadline. Stressful experiences often lead to what we want, or at the very least, they lead to the lesson we need.

Let's look at those two lists of emotions that you wrote down earlier. When you look at your list of feelings that you want to experience most days, was it all positive? Or did you list emotions like anxiety, stress, and concern? Did you realize that some of these "negative" feelings can actually produce positive results in your life? What if you flipped this script on your negative emotions and instead of avoiding them, you pursued them as a sign that you are on the right path like Ramit Sethi? In other words, what would happen if you put one of these negative feelings on the list of those you *want* to experience?

Using negative emotions to get to positive results is not the only benefit of experiencing negative emotions. Martin Luther King Jr. famously said in a speech about loving our enemies, "Darkness cannot drive out darkness; only light can do that. Hate cannot drive out hate; only love can do that." There is an inextricable link between positive and negative emotions. As darkness is the absence of light, many of the positive emotions in life have no context or meaning without their counterbalancing negative emotion.

For example, can we really know what joy is without experiencing deep sorrow? Possibly. Yet, once we experience great sorrow, we appreciate the times of deep joy much more. In other words, we cannot experience the full gamut of human emotion without experiencing the negative with the positive.

Experiencing a uniformly positive life is impossible. Some say life is 50% positive and 50% negative, even once we "make it." In fact, the great work to be done here isn't to avoid negative feelings, but to learn how to coexist with them, and to appreciate them while in their presence. This allows us to more fully experience the positive. However, this is not what most of us do when it comes to negative emotions. Instead, most of us attempt to resist or buffer these feelings.

## RESISTING, BUFFERING, AND ALLOWING NEGATIVE FEELINGS

Every year when the flu season nears, Kristen and I get our three children the flu vaccine. One year, when they were all under the age of nine, we scheduled our kids to get the shot at our pediatrician's office. Knowing that the flu shot has caused our kids some anxiety in the past, I thought it might be helpful to let them know what we were about to do. After setting the scene for them, we arrived at the doctor's office, and all three of my kids began to cry. Why? Because they were afraid, and the way that many children deal with fear is to resist it. In fact, during this specific episode, one of my kids tried to lock themselves in the bathroom so that they wouldn't have to get the vaccine. Resisting a negative emotion is akin to pushing against a door that someone else is attempting to open. We can white-knuckle our way through fighting a negative feeling—like fear in this flu shot example—when it arises, but all of us have a finite amount of willpower. It eventually runs out. This is the "fight" response of the fight-or-flight phenomenon.

The irony, of course, is that after my oldest kid, Grace, received her shot, she said, "That wasn't as bad as I thought it would be!" Yet, still, my two younger children kept screaming. It didn't matter that Grace told them it wouldn't be that bad. Just like it didn't matter when I told Grace the same thing before her shot. Wesley and Anna Ruth continued to resist their fear. After their shot was over, they had the same experience as Grace. It wasn't as bad as they thought it would be once it was over. In the end, resisting their fear for thirty minutes caused more agony than if they had just gone through the five-second experience of getting their flu shot. In a way, they were trading five seconds of future pain (the shot) for thirty minutes of guaranteed agony (the anxiety caused by their fear).

The point is that resisting our negative emotions is often worse than the experience itself. When we resist fear, impatience, anger, or sadness, it makes the situation worse. So if the "fight" response of the fight-or-flight phenomenon isn't the answer, maybe the solution is to avoid the negative experience by fleeing instead?

Some call the "flight" response "numbing." This is what people mean when they say they need something to "take the edge off." In coaching, we call this process buffering. Buffering is a means of reducing the psychological effects of a negative experience or emotion through our actions. For example, when the COVID-19 pandemic hit, I was already faced with running an online business at home in addition to my responsibilities as a husband, father of three kids who hate flu shots, and being a physician. Due to the pandemic, my three kids—aged nine, six, and three at the time—were suddenly all at home in virtual learning. This included being home on the days I would normally be working on The Physician Philosopher. Each day, I was now responsible for helping with homeschooling for Grace and Wesley while our threenager, Anna Ruth, yelled at me about wanting to do things by her own-big-girl-self. Hello, stress and anxiety!

At first, I tried white-knuckling it by resisting the stress. That lasted about a week. Then, there was no more fight left in my system. That's when I decided to flee the fight by numbing the pain through buffering. Most days by 3:00 p.m., I could be found making an old-fashioned with Bulleit Rye or pouring an IPA. I was using alcohol to buffer my stress. I wasn't working clinically on those days. Who cares if I drank a little to take the edge off, right? I would experience the stress of the day, feel the urge to drink, pop a cold one, and get the hit of dopamine from my limbic system that my body was craving. Then, I could escape for a little while. I wasn't alone in using alcohol to buffer this time either. In 2020, alcohol sales increased by 20% from March to September, according to a study published in the journal *Alcohol*.[31] Apparently, many of us used alcohol during the pandemic to cope.

My 3:00 p.m. drinking routine continued for a couple of months on the days that I was home until I realized this wasn't how I wanted to deal with anxiety or stress. I was buffering my stress and anxiety with alcohol. From our previous discussions, you will recall that our

---

31   João M. Castaldelli-Maia, Luis E. Segura, and Silvia S. Martins, "The Concerning Increasing Trend of Alcohol Beverage Sales in the U.S. during the COVID-19 Pandemic," *Alcohol* 96 (November 2021): 37–42, https://doi.org/10.1016/j.alcohol.2021.06.004.

circumstances do not determine our feelings, actions, or results. My drinking wasn't *caused* by the pandemic or being yelled at by my three-year-old. It was caused by how *I* decided to deal with my stress. My thoughts were the root cause of how I felt. My mind was telling me, *This is stressful. I just want this to go away.* So, I drank.

The problem here is that by buffering my negative feelings, I couldn't work through my anxiety and stress. It was the easy way out, and I was refusing to do the difficult thought work to find the root thought behind it all. What story was I telling myself about this situation? Why was it so hard? What was the actual problem? What thought was leading to all of this stress, and could I change the negative soundtrack that was running on repeat every day? Was there any way to lighten any of my responsibilities in my various roles as a doctor, dad, husband, and online entrepreneur? By drinking on those days, I was not doing the work. Fleeing the stress turned out to be much easier than fighting it.

Maybe you can't relate because alcohol isn't your go-to buffer. Not to worry. A lot of buffers exist. Other buffers include the following:

- **Overworking:** Staying at work longer to avoid the stress of going home. Whoever said medicine is stressful has never been a stay-at-home parent, apparently.
- **People-pleasing:** People-pleasing is much easier than working through the anxiety of having confrontational conversations with your boss, chair, partner, or colleague. I'd love to add that presentation you've asked me to do to my busy schedule so long as I don't have to argue about it.
- **Overeating:** Many of us turn to food to provide that hit of dopamine to escape our negative feelings. Don't tell me I can't have my cake and eat it, too. Those feelings aren't going to eat themselves!

- **Overspending:** Spending money when we feel discontent is common among doctors. I bet that new CT5-V Blackwing with the supercharged Corvette engine in it would make me happy. I mean, have you ever seen someone going zero to sixty in 3.5 seconds without a smile on their face?

- **Zoning out:** Many people use Netflix, Facebook, Twitter, or other entertainment and social media to avoid negative feelings like boredom or stress. There is no boredom that the infinite scroll on Facebook or a good Netflix binge can't fix!

- **Cell phones:** Likely the most common modern day buffer is cell phones. We use them as a way to escape from all sorts of situations. Picture a meeting before it starts. We could use that time to have an awkward conversation with our colleagues sitting around the table, or we could just mindlessly check the supercomputers in our pockets.

A buffer can be anything that gives us the ability to avoid negative feelings. Buffers are an escape mechanism. They are a way of fleeing from negative feelings. If you are using something to help you "take the edge off," "feel better," or "numb the pain," then it is most likely a buffer. While buffers may seem necessary for survival at times, they are always counterproductive in the long run. If we remember the motivational triad, it makes sense why we do this. Our brain is telling us to buffer because it is the most efficient way to avoid pain. When we feed that urge-desire-reward cycle, we condition a Pavlovian response to our buffers. Like the Group 2 German shepherds from Seligman's experiment, buffers become the lever we press when we get shocked in life. Helpful in the short-term, but it comes at great cost in the long run. Fortunately, there is a third option for working through our negative emotions—it is called allowing.

## ALLOWING INSTEAD OF RESISTING OR BUFFERING

When the COVID-19 pandemic hit, there were some free apps provided to healthcare professionals. One of the apps I downloaded during this time was a meditation app. I'll be the first to admit that meditation has never been my cup of tea, but I have found that over time it has proven helpful. My favorite kind of meditation involves a technique called "noting." When noting, the meditation instructor asks you to focus on something like your breathing. Over time, as you attempt to focus on your breathing, you will get distracted. The instructor knows this happens to everyone. And when we get distracted, this is when the instructor asks you to "note" whether that distraction is a "thought" or a "feeling." Once you have named the distraction a thought or a feeling, you are supposed to bring your focus back to your breathing. For example, when I am meditating, if I become distracted by the thought *Oh, yeah, I am supposed to record my next episode for* The Physician Philosopher *podcast; I wonder what I should talk about this week...* I may start thinking through what I want to say on the show, but eventually I will realize I am distracted from my meditation. When I become the watcher of my thoughts and realize I am distracted, my job is to note this as a distracting thought. Then, I bring my focus back to my breathing.

The reason that we are able to "note" during meditation is because humans have consciousness, which is the ability to be aware of our own thoughts and feelings. In other words, as human beings, we have the unique ability to be the watcher of our thoughts. In fact, the "real" person is not the thinker, but the watcher of our thoughts. Our consciousness is one of the characteristics that separates human beings from animals. When we utilize the process of noting during meditation, we become the watcher of our thoughts. This is how our consciousness is able to realize that we are distracted, to have self-compassion for becoming distracted (since it happens to us all), and to bring our focus back to our breathing. When we note something, we are neither trying to resist the distraction nor attempting to flee from it by using buffers.

The process of noting is exactly how "allowing" works, too. We do not have to "fight" our negative emotions by resisting them or fleeing from them through buffering or numbing. Instead, we can allow the emotion. Like a second person in the room, we can choose to watch our limbic system from our prefrontal cortex. We enter into our consciousness and become aware of our thoughts and feelings. If we have a bunch of kids screaming at home during a pandemic, this can lead to thoughts that then cause stress. When this happens, we can note the urge to drink without acting on it. We can sit with it. Describe it. Give words to the sensations these emotions produce. Then, once we note the stress, we can bring our focus back to our intentional decision not to drink. We aren't resisting the urge through white-knuckled willpower, which is a finite resource. We also aren't running from the stress by drinking an IPA. Instead, we are allowing it by noting it, and then coexisting with it.

If you are wondering how we might exercise this muscle of allowing negative emotions, it is the same way you might exercise any other muscle: repetition. A helpful exercise that we take many of our clients through is the process of explaining out loud how they feel. I'll ask them to imagine there is another person in the room who wants to understand how they feel. For example, I might ask the client I am working with to imagine explaining to my little boy, Wesley, what they are feeling. Imagine that Wesley heard you say that you were anxious, and he wants to know what anxiety is. What sensations does anxiety produce? How does it feel? Where in your body do you feel anxiety physically? They begin to describe the feeling as having a tightness in their chest, a racing heart, sweaty palms, and a clenched jaw. I then point out what Wesley likely would. Something like, "So, no one is trying to hurt you? They aren't trying to hit you? No one is chasing you with a gun or a knife? Your chest gets tight, your heart beats fast, your palms get sweaty, and you clench your teeth? That doesn't sound too bad."

By giving words to the physical sensations that our emotions produce, we are able to realize that the worst thing that can ever be caused by a negative feeling is...a feeling. Like with the noting technique in meditation, the process of allowing our negative feelings gives us the ability to realize that this terrible thing we are experiencing cannot cause us harm, unless we let it. No physical harm is going to come to us, no matter how hard our brain works to convince us otherwise. We can allow the anxiety without giving in to the desire and the dopamine hit we get from fulfilling that desire through buffering. And eventually, our circumstances will no longer trigger the urge to drink. It is a Pavlovian response. It can be unlearned and deconditioned with practice. Do this a hundred times, and you can diminish the response.

When we learn to allow our negative feelings, instead of resisting or buffering them, this lets us harness the power of negative feelings that produces positive results. It also allows us to have a full human experience where our negative emotions provide context to our positive emotions. With practice, allowing grants us the ability to reclaim autonomy over how we feel. With each step, we shift our continuum more and more toward becoming a self-determined physician working to enjoy this journey called life.

# CHAPTER 9

# Journey over Destination

"It is about the effort, not the outcome."
—A wise radiologist

PAUL WAS ON a run in Ardmore, the neighborhood surrounding the hospital where he was an anesthesiology resident at Wake Forest, when he came across an EMS team intubating a patient. As Paul stopped his run to watch what was quite a scene, he noticed that the EMS crew had performed an esophageal intubation on the patient. *This is what we call "tubing the goose" in anesthesia.* Recognizing the problem, Paul pointed it out to EMS. Naturally, the paramedics ignored the man in running shorts claiming to be a doctor. However, Paul felt obligated to act because it turns out that a breathing tube kills people when it isn't in the trachea. Knowing that this patient would die if EMS didn't remove the tube, Paul began to intercede. EMS wouldn't allow Paul to help, and that's when things got ugly. Because he interfered, the police placed Paul in handcuffs and threw him into the back of a cop car.

So, when someone at the North Carolina Society of Anesthesiologists (NCSA) meeting pointed Paul out to me, I had to meet him. Paul is an alumnus of the Wake Forest anesthesiology residency where I trained and where I still work as I write this book. Paul is a living legend. After walking over and introducing myself, I asked Paul if the story about getting arrested was true. He filled me in on all of the gory details (Paul had been right—the tube had been in the esophagus—and he did actually get arrested. Unfortunately, the patient didn't make it.) While the jail-time EMS story definitely lived up to the hype, it was not the story about being thrown in jail during residency that left the most indelible mark. Though, as an aside, Paul's short stint in jail prior to them confirming he was a physician and releasing him did impact the way I interacted with EMS a few years later, when I helped intubate a patient on the back of an EMS truck while on a family beach trip.

Instead, what stuck with me most from my conversation with Paul was a passing comment that he made about his time in Winston-Salem during medical school and residency at Wake Forest. The advice he imparted to me was this: "Jimmy, I know this part of life during residency seems hard. But if I am being honest, when I look back on that busy time in our tiny starter house in Ardmore while in Winston-Salem with my young family, it contains some of the happiest memories of my life."

The point he was trying to make was that life isn't all about getting to our goals. Sometimes, when we accomplish goals, like finishing training, things aren't always what we hoped they would be. In other words, Paul was encouraging me to enjoy the moment. To be present in it. To abide while in residency. I didn't believe him at the time.

*Surely, when I finish residency, fellowship will be better*, I thought. Yet I felt the same after it was done. *But wait, when I become an attending physician, I'll be much happier!* Nope. That didn't work either. *Wait, when I buy the big house or the 415HP rear-wheel-drive*

*Chevy SS that I waited a year to have shipped from Australia, that'll be the trick!* Not quite. As we previously discussed, this is called an "arrival fallacy." It's the idea that when we get to our goal, we will find long-lasting happiness. The happily-ever-after that we've read about in fairy tales.

Yet, if you are reading this book, I don't have to prove to you that it doesn't work like that. You likely have a life that many others in this world would envy. You are a physician who makes a very good paycheck. You work in a respected profession. Regardless of where you are in your journey, what you have achieved is impressive by any measure.

Yet, so many doctors aren't happy, despite all of this success. The satisfaction we receive from our goals can be short lived. Long-term satisfaction and contentment seem like the fountain of youth—impossible to find. So, if "getting there" isn't the answer, what is? That's the lesson Paul was trying to teach me. It is about being present in the moment. In the here and now. It is about enjoying the process of being who we are and who we are becoming. It is not about the destination. It is about the journey.

## THE PROCESS, NOT THE PRODUCT

While growing up, when we brought home report cards, my parents' focus was on us making good grades and making sure that we all lived up to our potential. To my parents, this meant getting As. Like most parents, their focus was on producing. My journey through medical school, residency, and fellowship continued that narrative. If I didn't make a certain score on my USMLE exam, I couldn't pursue the field I wanted. If I didn't receive honors on my third-year rotations, I was doomed to land in a mediocre residency program. If I failed in front of my attendings during residency, they'd think I was a bad resident. At least, these are the stories I told myself.

Not only did this perfectionism prevent me from learning from failure, but it also set up this narrative that accomplishments, awards, and accolades are the ultimate goal in life. The unintentional byproduct here is that perfection was required in order to feel worthy. Yet, what happens at the end of our training, when there are no accomplishments or awards left to win? For many doctors, they are left to practice medicine for the next twenty to thirty years, and to continually ask, "Is this really it? Is there no next step? If not, why am I so unhappy?"

This becomes a problem for many physicians who have learned to focus on accomplishments and arrivals in order to define their happiness and self-worth. Now, it isn't all bad having a focus on getting to our goals. For years, this goal-oriented nature is what got us through undergrad, medical school, and residency. The problem is what doctors do when the accomplishments and arrivals no longer exist.

Many of us turn into the walking examples of discontentment that Epictetus describes in a famous quote: "Nothing is enough for the man to whom enough is too little." That's how I felt. Like many hardworking doctors, nothing was ever good enough. I was a perfectionist (I'm now a recovering perfectionist). I would think things like: *I don't eat enough healthy food. I'm not patient enough with my kids. My business doesn't earn enough. I don't pursue my wife enough. My business isn't helping enough doctors. I'm not a good enough doctor. I don't make enough money.*

No accomplishment was ever enough. I was so focused on the end result that I couldn't enjoy the journey. Combine that with my goal-oriented nature, and I turned into a self-critical monster who was sapped of joy and contentment. Like many of the clients I would later coach, I was my own worst enemy. How did I get to this place where doing a good job was not enough? And who gets to decide what a "good job" or "enough" is anyway?

This focus on producing profoundly impacted my overall satisfaction and destroyed my sense of belonging, both at work and at home. I had fixed my gaze on the wrong goal. This realization came to a head during a coaching call with one of my clients, Simeon, a radiologist who suffered from an arrival fallacy, too. Simeon had multiple goals, which ranged from health and fitness goals to his career and home-life goals. Since he hadn't achieved his goals yet, he continually felt inadequate. Simeon told himself that until he reached his goals, he could not be happy.

I pointed out all the examples of things that Simeon had already accomplished and reminded him that before he accomplished them, he was sure they would make him happy. He then realized the truth. Even after all of his accomplishments, he wasn't happy. That's when Simeon realized life isn't really about getting "there." Instead, like Paul tried to teach me in residency, Simeon was coming around to the realization that life was more about the journey than the destination. That's when he said, "It is not about getting to my goals. It is about the effort, not the outcome." That thought stopped him in his tracks. To be honest, it stopped me in mine, too. What if we shifted the goal to be about our identity, the process, and the effort...instead of just the outcome? In other words, what if life was really about the process, not the product?

Imagine a world where our kids come home, and the question isn't about whether they got all As. Imagine a world where we ask them whether they put in the work, tried their hardest, and applied themselves. A world where parents compliment the hard-earned C as much as the hard-earned A. What lesson would this teach our kids about their self-worth, identity, and happiness in life, knowing that it comes from working hard and not from the end result and the never-ending need to produce? From this, they might learn the same lesson Kevin Durant's favorite quote teaches: "Hard work beats talent when talent fails to work hard."[32]

---

32  Most sources attribute this wisdom to high school basketball coach Tim

We can apply the same paradigm to our own life. We can learn to enjoy the process of hard work instead of continually setting our gaze on the goal that we want to achieve. That is exactly what I did when I set out to write this book. Instead of focusing on when the book would be done, I shifted my focus to enjoying the process of writing. The goal wasn't to be finished. It was to write. As Paul Valéry, the French poet, pointed out, "a work [of art] is never truly finished... but abandoned."[33] It is about the process, not the product. Those who are able to live in the moment understand this.

Now, hear me out. I am not saying that goal setting is bad. What I *am* saying is that focusing on the process over the end product has the potential to allow you to reclaim control over enjoying every moment of your journey. It increases both your personal and professional autonomy. It helps you feel like you belong as you take the same journey with others. And it certainly increases your ability to deal with the perceptions of failure.

When we move the goalpost to an indefinite point in the future, it has the potential to change everything. No longer is it about success or failure. No longer are we chasing a goal that inevitably leads to an arrival fallacy. Instead, the goal is to focus on who we are and who we are becoming. It puts us on a perpetual, never-ending journey that keeps us in the moment, which is when we are happiest.

In psychology, there is a name for the phenomenon of being caught up in the moment. It is called "flow." Flow was first described by Mihaly Csikszentmihalyi (pronounced "ME-HIGH CHICK SENT ME-HIGH"). It is the psychological state that occurs when we are deeply immersed in what we are doing. For writers, this happens when we write. Not when the book gets published. For athletes, this happens during the game, not when they win the

---

Notke, but Durant certainly helped popularize it.

33  Some have attributed this quote to E.M. Forster.

championship. For singers, this happens when they are singing, not after the concert is over. In other words, it happens during the journey, not when we get to the destination.

The video game *NBA Jam* understood the concept of flow when it famously said, "He's heating up," when a player was starting to get into the state of flow. And when the player was in a full-fledged flow state and couldn't miss, *NBA Jam* would loudly proclaim, "He's on fire!" We have other phrases for this in everyday speech, too. For example, we say things like "time flies when you are having fun" or in sports, we might say someone is "in the zone," "playing out of their mind," or "in the groove." My personal favorite, however, is when a broadcaster says an athlete is "unconscious" because they are playing so well.

When you step back and think about it, this is the same lesson Paul tried to teach me. That when we are in the process of living life, we are happiest. It is not when we finally get to our goals. Like the singer on stage, we are happiest when we are singing. This begs the question, then, why not focus on the writing of the book (instead of on finishing it)? Why not focus on training and playing the game (instead of on winning the championship)? Why not focus on being in the moment as a partner, parent, or physician (instead of focusing on when the next stage or life goal is met)?

Csikszentmihalyi says it this way in his seminal work called *Flow: The Psychology of Optimal Experience,*

> To overcome the anxieties and depressions of contemporary life, individuals must become independent of the social environment to the degree that they no longer respond exclusively in terms of its rewards and punishments. To achieve such autonomy, a person has to learn to provide rewards to herself. She has to develop the ability to find enjoyment and purpose regardless of external circumstances.

This thought process may sound familiar. Csikszentmihalyi's call to intrinsic motivation and autonomy comes from our internal perspectives and paradigms. Not the extrinsic rewards of our external environment. Csikszentmihalyi even mentions one of the ABCs of self-determination when he calls us to achieve autonomy. In a way, the point he makes is that contentment in life happens when we focus on internal rewards (i.e., enjoying the process) instead of being dependent on external rewards (i.e., the end product). Csikszentmihalyi calls us to realize that Deci and Ryan's autonomy happens when we focus on the internal process, not the external product.

This has the potential to impact everything. What if we shifted our goal away from getting to a certain weight on the scale and toward becoming someone who is on the journey to getting healthier? What if the goal wasn't to publish a bunch of papers but to be someone who researches and enjoys the process of learning and writing? What if our goal wasn't to run a marathon but to be someone who runs? What if our goal wasn't about determining what we want out of life but to simply be present in each and every precious moment that we have?

It turns out that when we shift the focus to the process, we take back our autonomy, which produces long-term satisfaction and contentment in life. As James Clear, the author of *Atomic Habits,* would say, "When you fall in love with the process rather than the product, you don't have to wait to give yourself permission to be happy."

When we shift our focus to the process, this shifts the questions we ask about life, too. No longer is the question "What do I want in life?" as we search for the missing ingredient that will magically make us happy. Instead, the focus becomes *the process* of becoming the sort of person we want to become in this world, and feeling more fully connected to a deeper sense of identity and purpose. At our core, who are we? Who do we want to be? What activities or events allow us to be "in the zone" or "in the groove?"

Answering these questions shifts our eyes to the process of becoming who we are and who we are working to become. Your goal might be to work on becoming a better mom or dad, or a better husband or wife. It could mean that you want to be a better teacher for your trainees, if you are an academic physician, or the best doctor you can be for your patients. Others might feel a deep longing to reconnect with their religious traditions. It is different for each of us, but the question is the same. Who do we want to be, and what do we want to do with this one amazing and crazy life we get on this earth?

As James Clear says, "Every action you take is a vote for the type of person you wish to become. No single instance will transform your beliefs, but as the votes build up, so does the evidence of your new identity."

Yet, this journey isn't for the faint of heart. What happens when we make a mistake along the way? When we don't show up as the best version of ourselves? When we have writer's block, scream at our kids, or make a mistake when taking care of a patient? The answer is that we learn how to choose curiosity over shame.

# Choosing Curiosity over Shame

"If you never know failure, you will never know success."
—Sugar Ray Leonard

IN 1976, TWO men met through a mutual friend. One was in high school. The other was in college at Cal Berkeley. The two of them would go on to pioneer one of the greatest companies ever created. After running the business for a time, they found great success. Yet, they realized that the two of them needed to hire someone to become the CEO of the company. This is when they decided to hire John Sculley away from PepsiCo with the famous line "Do you want to sell sugar water for the rest of your life? Or do you want to come with me and change the world?"

Steve Jobs was known for his visionary potential and ideas while Steve Wozniak was predominantly responsible for the engineering and integrating side of Apple. Given his visionary potential, you might wonder why Jobs didn't become the CEO himself at the time they hired John Sculley. We have to remember that Jobs founded

Apple after dropping out of college. He was young. Jobs also had a well-known penchant for being difficult to work with. He was demanding, blunt, and often rude. So, the investors and stakeholders of the company felt that he wasn't quite up to the task yet.

In fact, Steve Jobs was so challenging as a colleague that even after he created the first Macintosh, Jobs was ousted from his own business by the board of directors and current CEO. After what was a very public and humiliating dismissal, Jobs went on to build a new business called NeXT. He also founded Pixar during this time. After ten years of Apple's stock plummeting, NeXT would be acquired by Apple, and Jobs would be brought back into the fold by the company that fired him. Jobs would come to their rescue, and Apple would later achieve unprecedented success after creating iTunes, the iPod, and eventually the iPhone. Not too shabby for a company created by someone who never graduated from college.

However, I want to take you back. What if we didn't know the rest of the story? What if we put ourselves in Jobs' shoes the day he was fired and the ten years after where he was an outcast from the company he helped found? Can you imagine what that must have felt like walking in Steve Jobs' shoes? Many of us would have viewed ourselves as a complete failure, and fallen into the cognitive distortion we discussed previously of "shoulding ourselves into shame." Not Jobs, who famously said, "Getting fired from Apple was the best thing that could have ever happened to me. The heaviness of being successful was replaced by the lightness of being a beginner again. It freed me to enter one of the most creative periods of my life."

Do you see the beauty in that quote? Getting fired wasn't a failure at all. He viewed it the same way that Ramit Sethi did his failure file. It brought relief and opportunity. Jobs didn't stop there when he pointed out, "I've always been attracted to the more revolutionary changes. I don't know why. Because they're harder. They're much more stressful emotionally. And you usually go through a period where everybody tells you that you've completely failed."

Not only did Jobs refuse to accept failure and the shame that often comes along with it, but he also sought out the opportunities that caused stress and had the potential to fail. He wasn't alone. Sugar Ray Leonard captured this same sentiment in the quote at the beginning of this chapter: "If you never know failure, you will never know success." Success is on the other side of failure. Ryan Holiday, a modern-day stoic and author, teaches us the same idea in his book entitled *The Obstacle is The Way* when he points out that the obstacles we face in life are not *in* the way; they *are* the way to success. How, then, do we become like Jobs, Leonard, and Holiday and flip the script on failure? How can we learn to enjoy the process like Thomas Edison, who famously said, "I have not failed. I've just found 10,000 ways that won't work"? In order to answer this question, we must first talk about the reason none of us want to fail in the first place—shame.

## FLIPPING THE SCRIPT ON FAILURE

Doctors must be successful to get to where we are, which often means that we tend to be a bunch of overachievers, not failures. We view failure as something to be avoided, but have you ever thought about why? It all comes down to the second element of self-determination: our need to belong. When we fail, we face external criticism that can lead to shame and threaten our ability to feel like a valued member of the team.

Dr. Brené Brown—whom I introduced earlier in this book—says, "Shame is the most powerful, master emotion. It's the fear that we're not good enough." Shame attacks our sense of belonging. Shame thrives in isolation. It shifts our internal culture toward burnout and away from becoming self-determined. This is why it is such a deadly master emotion for burned-out doctors. When we feel like we aren't good enough or that asking for help is shameful and weak, self-determination isn't possible.

Shame leads to feeling unacceptable and unworthy, which has the potential to wreck any sense of belonging that we have worked to cultivate in our journey toward becoming self-determined physicians. Shame is also an indulgent emotion. Like overwhelm and worry, shame is never productive. It festers and grows in the darkness when we are too ashamed to share it. These are called indulgent emotions because they allow us to feel like we are doing something, when in reality, it is often easier to give in to it and produce a vicious cycle that prevents us from achieving the results we want in life. Just like eating multiple bowls of ice cream, it may feel good in the moment but likely doesn't lead to the results we want later.

In other words, shame is rarely helpful, and almost always counterproductive. Now, you might be asking, aren't we supposed to learn from our mistakes and mishaps like Steve Jobs, Sugar Ray Leonard, and Thomas Edison? This brings us back to our prior conversation about the difference between guilt and shame. When we look at the "Action" line and the "Results" line of our thought model (remember, CTFAR?), what is being produced? If it is positive or productive, it is likely a result of guilt, which often propels us to learn like Jobs, Leonard, and Edison. This might look like an apology to a loved one for something you said, or "making it right" as we say in our home. Perhaps it is a new experiment after learning your previous idea didn't work. Or learning to keep your hands up in a boxing match. If anything productive comes from what has happened, it is likely that guilt is driving your thought model.

On the other hand, if your end result is counterproductive, shame is likely the culprit. Let's say, for example, we are working to lose weight, and as a part of this, we have decided to forego dessert every day of the week except one cheat night on Fridays. Yet, we find that we are eating a bowl of ice cream on a Tuesday after a tough day at work. After we finish the dessert, an unintentional thought pops up: I can't believe I just did that. This is not going to help me lose weight. I am so fat. The thought (remember, it isn't the ice cream that produces your feelings...it is your thought about the ice cream) might lead to rumination about your apparent failure. Then, you question your resolve, and with the battle being lost, you find yourself going back for a second helping. This is a completely counterproductive thought model caused by shame. Not guilt.

You might not relate to this specific example. Regardless of your struggle, experiencing shame when we don't live up to our own expectations is universal. And the end result is always counterproductive.

Shame is never helpful or productive. Yet, it is an all too familiar feeling that haunts many of our worst days. The natural question is how do we defeat the shame that runs so rampant in our lives? How do we flip the script on failures and missteps when we have them? Is there a way to view our miscues as opportunities for improvements, like Jobs, Leonard, and Edison did, instead of letting them become perpetual generators of shame? Fortunately, the answer is yes.

## THE SHAME OF AN ENTREPRENEUR

It turns out that healthcare administrators aren't the only people who like to follow metrics. As a blogger in my early days, I did what every blogger does. I focused on The Physician Philosopher's page views as a sign of growth in the business. One day in 2018, I noticed a huge spike in traffic. So, I looked for the source of this traffic to see if I could replicate it in the future. It turned out that the source was coming from a social media mention on Twitter. Awesome, right?

The mention came from a blog post I wrote with some satire to my wife, Kristen, to inspire others to have a financial plan in place for those they love in case they die, particularly if their partner is not financially minded. The reason for this is that although some married couples share a love of personal finance, I've found that there is usually one person who is a much bigger money nerd than the other. In my marriage, the money nerd is me.

Kristen and I fill in each other's gaps extremely well. She is a detail-oriented person, and I am a big-picture abstract problem solver. She has a great memory and can read quickly. My nickname at work is Dory (yes, as in the forgetful fish), and I have a reading disability. (Who knew the words roll and role mean different things?) In fact, Grace, our 10-year-old, has been able to read faster than me since she was in fourth grade. Another difference between my wife and me is that I love talking and thinking about money, and Kristen hates it. So, while we have had a ton of conversations about the shared vision of where we want our life to go, Kristen trusts me to take care of the ones and zeroes when it comes to money. She has absolutely no interest in knowing what a Roth IRA is or the difference between a non-governmental 457 and a governmental 457.

With this background in mind, you'll understand what set the stage for the worst shame suckfest I've ever experienced as an entrepreneur. One that almost ended my online business and would have prevented me from ever writing this book. The post that was generating so much traffic included some inside jokes based on the information I just gave above, like the fact that I love money and have a reading disability while my wife has little interest in money and hates math. Apparently, it was frowned upon when I told Kristen she would have to do some math after I died in order to use the life insurance money she would receive. Without knowing the inside joke between us, the post was received poorly by an outside audience that didn't know either of our idiosyncrasies. Another reason for the response was that the audience was not familiar with personal finance writing, where math is always spelled out, no matter how simple.

To complicate matters, this audience also happened to be extremely feminist. When read through a feminist lens from someone that didn't know us, it came across as mansplaining and, I quote, "patriarchal bullshit." To them, I looked like a misogynist. That's when a physician picked it up and blasted it to their 300,000 Twitter followers. Hence the big blip in my traffic that day. While that traffic spike may have started with excitement, it ended in unadulterated shame.

The first comment I saw said, "Is it just me or is he making his death sound REALLY appealing?" My favorite one-liner, however, was this one: "Time for an attorney. The divorce kind." Apparently, the social media cancel-culture guidelines strictly state that when your spouse unintentionally puts their foot in their mouth, you have full right to murder or divorce them. Here I was thinking that I was glad I married a saint who could laugh at my stupid mistakes.

In total, there were more than 100 comments, many written by physicians calling for my death or divorce. I got absolutely blasted. Couple this with the fact that in real life—you know, the one that exists outside of social media comment sections—-I care deeply about women's rights and am a dad to two amazing girls (and an awesome little boy). Not to mention that I am married to a woman who is a far better human being than I am. The point is that all of these social media comments calling for my death or divorce hurt. A lot. They hit me where it mattered and shattered my sense of belonging. So, I went back and read my post through the same feminist lens as the commenters, and you know what? I realized that I had put my foot in my mouth more than once in the post I had written.

The problem wasn't the mistake, however. I could have looked at that mistake and chosen to improve through guilt. But I didn't choose guilt, which would have compelled me to do something good. Instead, I chose unadulterated shame that hurt for months. Like any person with a fierce need to belong, I wanted to make it right. So, I spent several hours writing a new post to explain the satire I had written in the original post, to apologize for some of it that came across as mansplaining, and to point out that asking for someone's death or divorce was harmful. By the way, whoever said "sticks and stones may break my bones, but words will never hurt me" was not only stupid, but wrong. Words hurt, if we let them.

The irony, of course, was that all of the people who destroyed me on social media likely never read the second post where I apologized. These keyboard warriors likely moved on to destroying someone else's life on social media. Another ironic thing about that post was that I received dozens of emails about that same letter from several of my readers (both men and women) who had discussions with their loved ones about their financial plan. In other words, the post accomplished its goal. Yet, it came at a great cost for me personally.

This cancel-culture experience taught me two important lessons that continue to serve me. I want to share them with you here. The first is this. In life, we can either be judged, or we can be ignored. It could be in an online patient review or a social media interaction gone awry like mine. However, in our polarized climate, it is impossible to avoid judgment. In fact, the only way to avoid it is to not put yourself out there, which means that you also miss serving all of the people who need your help but never knew you existed.

People will always have judgments and critical opinions about who we are, what we stand for, and the choices we make. Including people who are reading this book. So, if you haven't experienced judgment yet, it simply means that you haven't reached a large enough audience. But I bet you have experienced this sort of judgment and the accompanying shame. It might have been with a patient. Or a social media post or response. Or potentially even from a family member or friend. The fact is that even when we do everything right, we can be judged.

This brings me to the second important lesson, which is that we must learn how to deal with failure and the associated judgment and shame that come along with it. To do this, we must learn how to choose curiosity over shame.

## CHOOSING CURIOSITY

For a long time, I believed that it was my responsibility in life to provide grace, forgiveness, and compassion to others while having a perfectionist standard for myself. This is captured in a quote that used to be taped to my desk in residency. In it, Henry Ward Beecher says, "Hold yourself responsible for a higher standard than anybody else expects of you. Never excuse yourself. Never pity yourself. Be a hard master to yourself, and be lenient to everyone else."

While to this day I try not to pity myself—I believe self-pity is indulgent and counterproductive—the idea of being a hard master on myself and lenient to everyone else proved toxic. It makes the process of "becoming" impossible because none of us get it right every step along the way. This mindset has the potential to dismantle any sense of belonging we might have. In other words, I think Beecher was missing out on a key element, self-compassion.

Unlike Beecher, I now believe that with each decision we make, we are either moving toward or away from the kind of person we wish to become, and that we are more than any individual action or decision. We are a complicated mosaic working toward a goal. However, many of us view this journey toward self-improvement as a linear upward trajectory, like a line that always heads up and to the right at a forty-five-degree angle on the graph of our life's progress. Yet, that's not really how it works, and having that expectation produces a Beecher sort of mentality when our life veers off course.

Remember, our job is to cast as many votes as we can in the direction of the person that we are working to become. The point isn't to be a hard master with your mistakes or to avoid ever failing. It is about becoming better bit by bit so that one day we will be able to look up and see that we have become closer and closer to the sort of person we want to be.

While much of this work relates to the habits we choose that collectively work to create who we are and who we will be, an equally important work is how to handle the backward steps we will make while on this journey. Right now, you might be trying to change your eating habits, exercise more, correct your spending on Amazon, work on your ability to stand up for what you believe, get more sleep, journal more, pray more, or figure out how to get rid of that one bad habit.

In order to do this, we must have the ability to course-correct when we make a mistake. Just like Edison did when he invented the light bulb. Otherwise, our sense of belonging will be under attack. How do we treat ourselves when we have the bowl of ice cream or that beer we said that we wouldn't have? What do we do when we slip back into our impulsive behaviors and baseline habits? What do we do when we make a change at work and it doesn't pan out? Do we let the inner critic win? If you are a hardworking perfectionist like me, the answer is likely yes. But it doesn't have to be this way.

I once had a client who decided he was going to start eating better. Let's call him John. Consciously, John made the decision to have a healthier lifestyle for himself and his family. Yet, every time someone put food in front of him, he felt like he couldn't help but eat it.

John consistently found himself eating out of habit and seemingly without thought. His unintentional model was a result of having an urge to eat, filling that desire, and getting the hit of dopamine that accompanied a mouth full of pizza. We did the work to intentionally choose what he ate twenty-four hours in advance, which studies have shown improves your chances of success. However, an equally important work was helping John be kind to himself when he slipped back into his old ways. That's when we taught John to choose curiosity over shame. Instead of fat-shaming himself with how bad he was and how he couldn't believe he slipped into his old routine, he changed his internal narrative by asking questions.

Out of a place of self-compassion, John learned how to choose curiosity instead of shame. To do this, John learned how to become curious about his choices. Was there anything that went well that he could praise himself for? What was the situation when he decided to eat that slice of pizza? Could he avoid that situation in the future? If not, how could he set himself up better for success? What could he do differently next time? Was there something he could learn from this experience?

You'll notice immediately that this turns John's unintentional and judgmental lower brain off and it turns his *intentional* problem-solving brain on. In the words of Tversky and Kahneman, curiosity makes this a methodical System 2 thought process instead of a judgmental and automatic System 1 thought process. When he chose curiosity, John was able to remove tempting food from his house in order to make doing the right thing easier. He decided to make a meal plan to give himself a better chance of sticking to eating the right thing. And he also asked for some accountability from his family.

The point is that choosing curiosity and answering the questions that curiosity produces turns our unproductive shame into a productive curiosity. It allows us to continue the back-and-forth journey required to get to our goals. It allows us to remain goal-oriented while also allowing us to course-correct without stumbling through shame. Instead of choosing shame, we have the opportunity to think, *Huh, that's interesting...I wonder why I did that.* In other words, we can *learn* like Jobs, Edison, and Sugar Ray Leonard instead of judging it and producing the counterproductive shame spiral I experienced from my viral blog post. If shame thrives in silence and produces inaction, then curiosity and talking about it is the antidote.

You may already be familiar with this idea of curiosity from aviation and medicine. This process is called a debrief, which is used to identify problems and areas of improvement. Debriefs start out asking about what went well. Then, the attention is turned to what didn't go well and why. And finally, the team discusses what they could do differently next time. When we debrief, instead of pointing fingers while we shame and blame others, the team can move forward and be better the next time, all without sacrificing the team's sense of belonging. When we choose curiosity over shame in our personal lives, the same process unfolds. We are choosing systematic improvement instead of a shameful attack on our inner sense of belonging.

Steve Jobs spoke about his firing from Apple, the company he founded at the age of twenty, and his associated public failure in a now-famous Stanford commencement speech in 2005.

> What had been the entire focus of my adult life was gone. And it was devastating. I didn't really know what to do for a few months. I felt like I had let the previous generation of entrepreneurs down—that I had dropped the baton as it was being passed to me. I met with David Packard [of Hewlett-Packard] and Bob Noyce and tried to apologize for screwing up so badly. I was a very public failure, and I even thought about running away from [Silicon] valley...I had been rejected, but I was still in love...I didn't see it then, but getting fired from Apple was the best thing that could ever have happened to me.[34]

Jobs felt guilt from what he had done, and then became curious about how he could mend his broken situation. In the same Stanford commencement speech Jobs ends by saying, "For the past thirty-three years, I have looked in the mirror and asked myself, 'If

---

34  "Steve Jobs' 2005 Stanford Commencement Address," YouTube, March 7, 2008, https://www.youtube.com/watch?v=UF8uR6Z6KLc.

today was the last day of my life, would I want to do what I am about to do today?' And whenever the answer has been 'no' for too many days in a row, I know I need to change something."

When you notice that you are casting too many votes in a direction that you don't want for too many days in a row, I hope that, like Steve Jobs, you wield the power of guilt in order to make the change you know you need. And when, like Jobs, you make a mistake along the way, I hope that you learn how to choose curiosity and the self-compassion that accompanies it.

# CHAPTER 11

# The Lost Art of Self-Compassion

"Self-care is not selfish. You cannot pour from an empty vessel."
—Eleanor Brown

LONG BEFORE TAMPING and boring machines, railroad workers used thirteen-pound tamping rods to place gunpowder into holes in order to build railroad tracks. With the rod, they would place a small amount of gunpowder into the hole before it was ignited in order to clear the way for the track. This was something that Phineas Gage had done on numerous occasions, but on September 13, 1848, something went wrong. This time when Gage put his tamping rod into the hole to load the gunpowder, it ignited prematurely. His tamping rod suddenly launched backward with strong force. The damage was immediate as the tamping rod went through Gage's skull and into his left frontal lobe.

After surviving his accident, Gage experienced major personality changes. His social filter disappeared, and Gage was subsequently known for his foul language and random outbursts in public. In fact, those that knew him before and after the accident said that the Phineas before the accident was not the same person as the man they experienced after. Gage's injury with a tamping rod is what led to some of the medical community's initial understanding about the function of the frontal lobe, which is responsible for personality and executive decision-making.

Phineas Gage is not alone, however, in his traumatic brain injury. Many patients have had a lesion on their brain in a variety of locations that have produced equally interesting phenomena. Each lesion has allowed us to better understand the anatomic responsibility of the human brain. One such phenomenon is called anosognosia, a condition in which patients have a very powerful form of neglect. In fact, it is such a powerful form of neglect that patients who suffer from anosognosia are completely unaware of their disability. For example, patients with anosognosia may be totally blind, yet refuse to acknowledge their blindness despite overwhelming evidence. They will deny their disability despite running into walls, not flinching when a fist is thrust toward their face, and having no reaction to bright lights. Anosognosia is sometimes accompanied by the more typical presentation of neglect, too, where a patient denies that their body parts are their own.

Unlike the changes in decision-making and personality that Gage experienced due to damage to his frontal lobe, anosognosia typically comes from damage to the nondominant side of the brain (the right side for most). Specifically, a lesion to the parietal lobe or a larger lesion that interrupts the frontal-temporal-parietal area.

It was in a 1999 study entitled "Unskilled and Unaware of It: How Difficulties in Recognizing One's Own Incompetence Lead to Inflated Self-Assessments" that researchers observed an interesting phenomenon that they would dub "the anosognosia of everyday

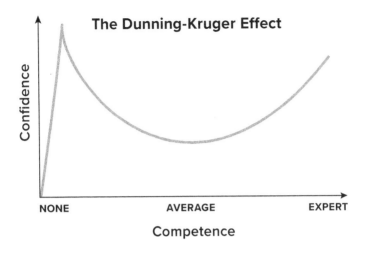

The Dunning-Kruger Effect

life."[35] This is the phenomenon that happens when "you don't know what you don't know." Or as Charles Darwin put it, this is when "ignorance more frequently begets confidence than knowledge."

This 1999 study was performed by two researchers named David Dunning and Justin Kruger, which is why the effect they described is now famously called the Dunning–Kruger effect. The Dunning–Kruger effect is the cognitive bias or thought error that occurs when people overestimate their knowledge or confidence in a given area relative to objective criteria. The idea is best captured in their now-famous Dunning–Kruger curve shown here:

On the x-axis is competence (which is sometimes labeled "experience"). On the y-axis is confidence. While most people likely assume that their confidence and competence increase linearly with experience, that is not how it actually works. And this is an

---

35  Justin Kruger and David Dunning, "Unskilled and Unaware of it: How Difficulties in Recognizing One's Own Incompetence Lead to Inflated Self-Assessments," Journal of Personality and Social Psychology, 77, no. 6, 1121–1134, https://doi.org/10.1037/0022-3514.77.6.1121.

important realization for burned-out doctors looking to master the competence found in Deci and Ryan's model of self-determination. What actually happens during the learning process is that most people experience a large increase in their confidence as their competence grows as a novice. I distinctly remember this point in training after my first year learning anesthesia in residency. At first, everything required effort. By the end of the year, however, I felt pretty proficient and confident in my abilities. My confidence increased in lockstep with my competence until I was overconfident. I had arrived at the peak shown on the left of the Dunning–Kruger curve, which is affectionately known as "Mount Stupid." This is the point at which we don't know what we don't know.

Not to worry, this moment would be short lived as I became a PGY-3, a year known for being a humbling crucible. I spent each of the first six months of my PGY-3 year in a subspecialty I had not yet experienced. By the end of that year, I had swiftly descended Mount Stupid, where my confidence would hit rock bottom. The bottom of this curve in medicine is when, I believe, doctors experience their first run-in with imposter syndrome. It is at this point that many doctors feel like frauds waiting to be caught. Their competence and experience have increased, but their confidence has been destroyed.

Fortunately, this usually recovers by the end of training. At this point, doctors feel pretty good about their skillset and what they are able to accomplish. Yet, this isn't the end of the imposter syndrome journey. In fact, I think the Dunning–Kruger curve shown above doesn't quite depict the doctor's journey in medicine. Based on my experience working with physicians who struggle with imposter syndrome as attending physicians, the curve actually looks more like this:

You'll notice that as we near the end of training, doctors feel pretty good about their skillset. Yet, when we are in our first few months of being an attending physician, many doctors quickly transition into the classic "fake it 'til you make it" phenomenon, and

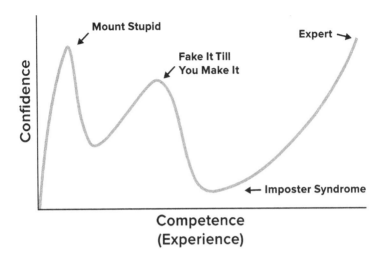

their confidence again dips for a time. The reason for this is that doctors cannot see absolutely everything the world of medicine has to offer during training. The practice of medicine is an ever-changing journey as medical knowledge improves and we gain experience seeing things we have not come across before. As this happens, we slowly slip from "fake it 'til you make it" into the abyss. It may be due to a mistake, a missed read, or a bad patient outcome or review. As compassionate physicians, we feel responsible, and as these negative experiences add up, we eventually fall into full-fledged imposter syndrome.

The peak of my imposter syndrome happened during a Level 1 trauma case early in my career as an attending physician. I was on second shift, which is often the busiest shift from start to finish for anesthesiologists at Wake. The story relayed to my team when the patient arrived was that the patient was a teenage kid who had been trying to score some weed but had instead been badly injured with a GSW (gunshot wound) to the abdomen. Initially, the patient presented to an outside hospital where the emergency room doc put a large central line into their right subclavian, started giving blood products, and then sent the patient to us while on vasopressors because we were the closest Level 1 trauma center.

By the time the patient arrived in our operating room, the patient had already received multiple units of blood, was intubated, and was on vasopressors through the subclavian central line the outside ED had placed. However, the patient didn't have an arterial line, and his noninvasive blood pressure cuff was taking longer and longer to measure. This kid was continuing to circle the drain. That's when I noticed the silence, the most alarming sound in all of anesthesia. During a trauma, silence is a bad omen, whether it is a Yankauer that doesn't make a noise when it is sucking vast amounts of blood or the silent cycle of a blood pressure cuff that won't provide a number because the patient's blood pressure is too low to measure. This patient would experience both forms of silence. Given this patient's vasopressor requirement, it was challenging to get an arterial line placed so that we could better monitor his hemodynamics. Multiple team members attempted to place the arterial line while I was directing the patient's care. That's when I decided to step in.

As an anesthesiologist with a fellowship in regional anesthesia, I have to be extremely proficient with ultrasound-guided procedures. So, I grabbed an ultrasound and worked hard to place a left-sided radial and eventually brachial arterial line (the surgeons would attempt to place a femoral as well, which proved unhelpful given the injury we would later find). It was at this time that I experienced my first fixation error as an attending physician. Having lost the view of the forest for the trees, I was no longer in charge of the patient's care. Instead I focused on the individual tree, the arterial line placement. The noninvasive blood pressure cuff cycled more than once without producing a blood pressure (a sign that the blood pressure isn't high enough to measure); the end tidal $CO_2$ was dropping as well (another sign that adequate perfusion is no longer happening); and the patient was about to code. I hadn't noticed any of this until one of my anesthesiology partners, who had snuck into the room during all the commotion, spoke up. "He is about to code. Start doing compressions." Moments later, the patient lost a pulse. We never got it back.

My partner, who helped me during the case, was kind enough to debrief with me after the patient died, and he told me, "Jimmy, it is our job to keep the big picture in view until we can't anymore. You got fixated on the arterial line. Next time, try not to lose the forest for the individual trees." It turned out that my fixation error didn't matter because the bullet had obliterated a portion of the patient's inferior vena cava and aorta, which explained why our massive transfusion didn't make a dent despite large-bore access and multiple rapid transfusers. We could not keep up with the blood loss.

While the injury wasn't survivable, I learned a lesson that day: fixation errors can be deadly. When we focus on a symptom and not the diagnosis, it can cause real harm. This error sent me reeling. Here I was as a young attending physician, and I felt like I had let my team down. I talked with the anesthesia residents I worked with in the case to make sure they were okay. Seeing the loss of a young life is hard to process. I knew how they were feeling, because I felt it, too.

We discussed what went well, what did not, and what we could have done differently. After listening to their perspectives first, I reassured my trainees that there was little we could have done in this case given the extent of the injury this patient had sustained. I pointed to it as an opportunity to learn. We discussed the emotional response they felt, and I reminded them that this was evidence that they were caring and compassionate physicians. I told them, "Keep your heads up! You did a fantastic job. I would absolutely let you take care of me in my moment of greatest need."

Yet, if I am being honest, I was a total hypocrite. My inner dialogue told me that my fixation error was unacceptable. I lost sleep over the error, let it lead to shame, and generalized this cognitive error into meaning I was a bad anesthesiologist. Just like I had with the central line mistake I made during my intern year. While I told my residents to brush it off and to keep their heads up, I felt like a total imposter waiting to be caught. I felt like a fraud. This began my descent into the lonely second valley of the medical Dunning–Kruger curve drawn above. I was journeying into full-fledged imposter syndrome. My perfectionist tendencies didn't allow me to make an error without my Henry Ward Beecher inner self-critic coming out. Instead, I chose to internalize my shame and suffer in silence.

## THE SYNERGY OF IMPOSTER SYNDROME AND BURNOUT

Dr. Christina Maslach, the creator of the Maslach Burnout Inventory, and Dr. Michael P. Leiter describe burnout as "a psychological syndrome emerging as a prolonged response to chronic interpersonal stressors on the job." They go on to say that "the three key dimensions of this response are an overwhelming exhaustion, feelings of cynicism and detachment from the job, and a sense of ineffectiveness and lack of accomplishment."[36] This definition includes "a sense of ineffectiveness and lack of accomplishment," which ought to sound very familiar in our current discussion on imposter syndrome. It sure sounds like the language of the fraud, feeling ineffective with our skills and ignoring our accomplishments while we focus instead on what has gone wrong. Unfortunately, it is relatively common, too, with some studies suggesting that the rate of imposter syndrome ranges from as low as 20% to as high as 60% of all physicians.[37]

---

36 Christina Maslach and Michael Leiter, "Understanding the Burnout Experience: Recent Research and its Implications for Psychiatry," *World Psychiatry* 15, no. 2 (2016): 103–111, https://doi.org/10.1002/wps.20311.
37 Gottlieb, "Impostor Syndrome," *Medical Education*, https://doi.org/10.1111/medu.13956.

Given that imposter syndrome directly attacks our perceived competence, one of the key components of self-determination, it makes sense that there would be a relationship between imposter syndrome and burnout. In fact, Gottlieb and colleagues found in their literature review published in *Medical Education* that imposter syndrome was linked to higher rates of burnout and suicide among both practicing physicians and physicians-in-training. Gottlieb also found higher rates of imposter syndrome in bad medical cultures and in physicians with low self-esteem.

For most of my life, I viewed self-esteem (or self-confidence) as virtually identical to confidence, arrogance, and pride. However, during coaching certification, I was introduced to the concept of how self-confidence and confidence differ. Confidence has the typical connotation most of us would apply to these words. The Google dictionary defines confidence as "a feeling of self-assurance arising from one's appreciation of one's own abilities or qualities." Said differently, confidence is the self-assurance we bring to the table when we have done something hundreds or thousands of times. Confidence is what a big-leaguer stepping to the plate experiences when he knows that he can hit a baseball because he has done it thousands of times before.

Self-confidence, however, arises from a deeper sense of identity about who and what we are, apart from our accomplishments and experiences. Unlike confidence, which comes from experience, as depicted in the Dunning–Kruger curve, self-confidence comes from a deep-rooted sense of identity. It is knowing who and what we are, apart from what others say, our public accomplishments, or the number of times that we have done something. In a sense, self-confidence is internal, whereas confidence is external.

While a physician may have loads of confidence in a skill that they have completed hundreds or thousands of times, we can simultaneously have very little self-confidence. Said differently, it is possible for a physician to trust their skills due to experience and repetition at the same time that they think they are not a very good doctor due to low self-esteem and lack of self-confidence. When low self-esteem is present, imposter syndrome is sure to follow.

So, what did the authors of the *Medical Education* literature review say had the potential to improve imposter syndrome? First, they detailed how personal and group reflections provided benefits. This may explain why physicians who go through individual and group coaching have been shown to have decreased burnout and emotional exhaustion, and improved quality of life.[38] If we look back at the ABCs of the self-determined physician, these physicians thrive when they feel a deep sense of community and belonging, where they can be themselves. Sharing lived experiences with other physicians on the same journey can help foster that goal. Further, the authors of the *Medical Education* article argued that validating success, social support, and positive affirmations improved imposter syndrome as well.

This is worth mentioning because positive affirmations, or the process of reminding yourself of the beliefs you choose to hold as true, is exactly what we have discussed in this book. This is the same process that Covey, Mandela, and Rosa Parks exemplified. And it is the same tradition that arises from Epictetus, the Serenity Prayer, and coaching. Choosing to affirm what you believe about who and what you are can prove powerful in your fight against imposter syndrome. Having friends and colleagues around that will do the same also provides a tremendous amount of help. However, it is equally important to learn how to harness this skill within ourselves and provide the same comfort to ourselves that we would to a friend.

---

38  Liselotte Dyrbye et al., "Effect of a Professional Coaching Intervention on the Well-being and Distress of Physicians: A Pilot Randomized Clinical Trial," *JAMA Internal Medicine* 179, no. 10 (October 2019): 1406–14, https://doi.org/10.1001/jamainternmed.2019.2425.

## SELF-COMPASSION

Previously, we discussed that the word compassion is composed of two roots—*pati* which means "to suffer" and *com* which means "with." Compassion is usually considered an outward projection toward other people. In other words, compassion means to suffer with someone else. However, that is not the only way to utilize compassion. We can also direct it internally. This iteration is called self-compassion.

Dr. Kristin Neff, a psychologist, researcher, and author of the book *Self-Compassion*, argues that self-compassion is composed of three parts: self-kindness, common humanity, and mindfulness. Self-kindness is an ability to look at ourselves from an objective third-person perspective. For example, we might look at our situation and what has just happened and find ourselves being self-critical. After my arterial line fixation error, that's exactly what I did. I couldn't believe what I had done. I told myself that my fixation clearly meant I did a bad job taking care of that patient. Yet, I didn't have to listen to that inner critic. Instead, when I talked about it with one of my other friends after the event, I realized that a fixation error is something that everyone experiences, and this allowed me to be a little kinder toward myself. It allowed me to cozy up to the fire of self-kindness on what had otherwise felt like a pretty cold and dreary day.

Later on, I learned that I could use this skill even when I didn't have a chance to talk with someone else. It is a skill I could employ when I drank one more beer than I "should" after a tough day. Or when I raised my voice at my kids after the thirteenth time they asked me to buy them a cell phone. I could even use this skill when I had a hard time writing this chapter the first time I sat down to write it (*true story)*!

How can we employ this skill? By asking ourselves a simple question. If someone else was going through the same thing that we are going through, what would we say to them?

For example, what would I say to a friend who had two beers instead of one after a bad day at work? *I'd tell them that we all need to take a load off sometimes. I'm just as guilty as the next.* What would I tell them if they raised their voice after having to say the same thing over and over to their kids? *I would probably tell them that they're a human having a human experience, and that their kids need to see them fail so that they can see what repentance, forgiveness, and reconciliation look like.*

Answering the question of what we would say to someone else going through a similar situation as ours makes it much easier to have compassion toward ourselves. It helps us silence that perfectionistic inner critic. This first element of self-compassion is unfortunately rare in the physician world, yet self-kindness is a learned skill that we develop in group coaching settings all the time.

The second aspect of self-compassion, Neff points out, is captured in our common humanity. In other words, it is the idea that we are human, and "to be human is to err." I often capture this sentiment with my residents after they make a mistake and I see that they are beating themselves up for it. In this setting, I'll often turn to them and sarcastically say, "You know, I've never made a single mistake in my life." After they laugh, I usually follow that up with, "You know what you can learn from me? If an imperfect guy like me can be a good anesthesiologist, then so can you. Keep your head up. We learn through mistakes and failure. This is a good thing."

Speaking this way provides a lethal blow to the perfectionist tendencies that cause our imposter syndrome. We all make mistakes, each and every day. We have survived 100% of our bad days, and if we are being honest, the bad days are the days that we usually learn the most. So, when we take part in the shared consciousness and experience of being human, we can have a little more self-compassion after having a human moment of error, including when we fail. Learning this helps us embrace the lessons we learned earlier in this book from Thomas Edison, Ramit Sethi, and Sugar Ray Leonard.

The third component of self-compassion is equally important—and just as lacking—in the physician community: being mindful. In coaching, we call the process of being mindful "holding space" for a client. Holding space means serving as a nonjudgmental mirror for someone else. When someone holds space for us to be human, we can acknowledge that life can be hard. Then, we can work through it by allowing the negative feelings that often result.

In practice, this might look like admitting that things are difficult sometimes. Mindfulness is not about negating the feeling or trying to escape from it. We have already discussed that resisting and buffering our negative emotions is unhelpful. Instead, being mindful gives us the ability to allow a negative feeling and to treat ourselves with the same kind of empathy we would give someone else. Think about it. If a friend told you that they missed a diagnosis on a challenging patient, would you look at them and say, "You must be a terrible physician?" Of course not. Instead, you would provide a much more mindful comment like, "Man, that sucks. I've totally had something like that happen before." Acknowledging that life is not always cheery is half the battle. As we have previously discussed, this is not something we even want. Negative emotions and feelings serve an important role in our life. Being mindful of their existence allows us to step into this truth.

Historically, self-compassion has not come easily to physicians. Fortunately, like any other skill, self-compassion is something we can hone with practice. In the same way we learned how to perform a physical exam or to operate, we can learn how to wield self-compassion with consistent and steady use. However, in order to truly understand self-compassion, we must do more than understand what compassion looks like. We must also spend time understanding what the word "self" means.

## IDENTITY WORK

Self-compassion is key in the fight to defeat imposter syndrome and to produce the confidence and competence of a self-determined physician. However, it is not the only work to be done. According to the source of all knowledge and wisdom (a.k.a. Wikipedia), "Impostor syndrome (also known as impostor phenomenon or impostorism) is a psychological occurrence in which an individual doubts their skills, talents, or accomplishments and has a persistent internalized fear of being exposed as a fraud."[39]

The work to be done with imposter syndrome involves more than learning how to forgive ourselves when we make mistakes. While self-compassion is key, if we are going to shift our continuum toward self-determination, we must also recognize our competence even when others might not. In other words, in order to defeat imposter syndrome and avoid feeling like a fraud, we must replace this feeling with a deep-seated sense of knowing who we are. Are we really trying to pull the wool over the eyes of those around us? Are we unjustifiably claiming accomplishments or recognition that we don't deserve? The answer for all of the hardworking physicians reading this book is almost certainly "no."

One useful exercise that we can employ to defeat this narrative of being a fraud is to separate fact from fiction. On one coaching call, I was talking with Kisha, a surgeon. Kisha had a bad patient outcome, so she was doubting her surgical and decision-making abilities. Her patient experienced poor wound healing that required multiple operations, and so Kisha was beating herself up because she felt like the patient's outcome was her responsibility.

This is an easy narrative to assume, because any good physi-

---

39  Wikipedia, s.v. "Impostor syndrome," last modified May 10, 2022, 16:44, https://en.wikipedia.org/wiki/Impostor_syndrome.

cian feels responsible for the outcomes of their patients. Yet, that does not mean that every outcome is the physician's fault, which is what Kisha was telling herself. She felt like a fraud. That was until we helped her take her blinders off by separating the facts from her story. In other words, we discussed the salient details of Kisha's surgical case that any two people would agree on as circumstantial facts, and separated those from the story she was telling herself about those facts.

It turns out in this situation, her patient came in with a head and neck malignancy that required an operation, had poorly controlled diabetes with an elevated hemoglobin A1C, obesity, and a penchant for smoking. Given the cancer diagnosis, there wasn't a way to properly optimize this patient prior to the surgical procedure. Waiting was not an option. During the case, Kisha asked for a second opinion from a colleague, who agreed with her assessment and course of action. Despite all of this, the patient ended up having poor wound healing that led to multiple surgical procedures.

I wrote down the details of Kisha's story and then shared the facts back to her. I asked her what she would think of a colleague who did all of the things that she had done. Kisha said, "It sounds like they took really good care of the patient." It turns out that this surgeon's imposter syndrome was not a result of a lack of skill, accomplishment, or education. Instead, Kisha's imposter syndrome was caused by her narrative that a bad outcome meant she hadn't done a good job. While coaching is one of the quickest ways to work through a bad case of imposter syndrome, you can also learn to do this work by yourself.

The next time you doubt your decisions, suffer from imposter syndrome, or have trouble sorting through your thoughts, write them down. This is called a thought download, and here is how it works.

First, take five to ten minutes and write down everything that comes to mind about the situation you are working through. Don't limit or censor what comes out onto the paper (or keyboard). Just write. After you perform your thought download, come back and read what you have written. Circle or underline the facts in the case, remembering that a fact is something two lawyers would agree on in court. Facts are objective and verifiable. Everyone would agree with them. For example, "I did a bad job" is not a fact. "The patient underwent multiple operations" is. Finally, take stock of the amount of your thought download that is a story, and not a fact.

When you go through this exercise, you might note how very few facts there are, and how the vast majority of what you have written is your narrative, perspective, paradigm, or story about those facts. These narratives are the gaps we fill in with the few facts we have. And your narrative is up to you, my friend. You can choose to keep it and learn to allow the feeling that your thought is producing, or you can choose to change it if that thought is not serving you.

This process of sorting out fact from fiction—whether with an objective third party like a coach who is holding space for us or with our own pen and paper—helps us to have self-compassion. It allows us to suffer with ourselves in the same way we would with a friend. This works against the Dunning–Kruger curve and allows doctors to increase the perceived competence and reduce the lack of accomplishment seen in burned-out doctors. In order to do this, however, we must learn how to say no to the fraudulent narratives we tell ourselves so that we can say Hell Yes to what matters most.

# CHAPTER 12

# The Hell Yes Policy

"Remember that if you don't prioritize your life, someone else will."
—Greg Mckeown

BILL GATES, THE founder and visionary leader of Microsoft, is well known for taking two separate one-week breaks from his normal work schedule to have "think weeks." During each of these seven-day think weeks, he would disconnect from technology and other commitments, and you guessed it, he would *think*. He would arrive either via seaplane or helicopter. With him on his air transport of choice, Gates would bring multiple boxes of reports written by Microsoft employees pitching new ideas and innovations. Some accounts of these think weeks say that Gates would spend more than fifteen hours each day reading through these innovative ideas. So much for taking a "break," huh?

Gates recognized that without dedicated time to consider novel ideas for Microsoft, innovation was unlikely to happen. There is always another fire to put out as a leader of a company or organization. It was during these think weeks that Gates came up with the ideas for Microsoft's Tablet PC, and also Internet Explorer, which dominated the scene as the preeminent web browser of the 1990s and early 2000s.

Bill Gates knew that time to think was a top priority. He understood what Stephen Covey meant when he said, "The key is not to prioritize what's on your schedule, but to schedule your priorities." Covey also quipped that "The main thing is to keep the main thing the main thing."

If many of the top thinkers have underscored the importance of prioritizing our priorities and mastering our schedule instead of letting our schedules master us, why then do so many physicians struggle to find the time they need to complete what is most important to them? What Gates and Covey knew, and what so many hardworking doctors are learning, is that our calendars must reflect our priorities and that this won't happen by accident. Greg McKeown, the author of *Essentialism*, drives this point home when he teaches us where the origin of the word priority came from in the first place. McKeown explains,

> The word priority came into the English language in the 1400s. It was singular. It meant the very first or prior thing. It stayed singular for the next five hundred years. Only in the 1900s did we pluralize the term and start talking about priorities. Illogically, we reasoned that by changing the word we could bend reality. Somehow we would now be able to have multiple 'first' things. People and companies routinely try to do just that.
>
> One leader told me of this experience in a company that talked of 'Pri-1, Pri-2, Pri-3, Pri-4, and Pri-5' [demarcating priorities 1 through 5]. This gave the impression of many things being the priority but actually meant nothing was.

This misunderstanding about priorities is not unique to business. Sarah was an emergency medicine physician and leader in her department. She was also a coaching client of mine, and on this particular call, Sarah wanted to discuss the difficulty she had getting things done that were important to her. So, I asked, "How do you go about planning your week?"

Sarah explained that she looked at her calendar to see the commitments and obligations that had already made their way onto her calendar. The good doctor then added other items to her agenda as they came up. Then, she spent the remainder of her time putting out the fires that inevitably came up. What she discovered was that there wasn't enough time in the day to get everything done. After this happened for months on end, things like exercise, eight hours of sleep, and date nights with her husband rarely made it onto the calendar.

This is what happens when we spend our time dealing with urgent tasks regardless of their importance. We must answer the email, we must attend the surprise meeting, and that new lab result or patient message surely isn't going to answer itself! All of these tasks are not intrinsically evil. Although I know a physician or two who might want to debate me on that. However, all of the fires that doctors continually put out are an attack on personal autonomy and time. When our personal autonomy is not a stronghold, the ever-elusive work-life balance that so many doctors want feels like a pipe dream. There are two lessons here. This is the first:

When you say yes to one thing, you are often saying no to what matters most.

So, before you say yes, consider whether the new opportunity is worth the cost. When we spend most of our time putting out fires, this is when our schedule has the propensity to master us. It is an insidious march toward the unintentional life that seems to happen *to* us instead of *for* us. In order to protect what matters most in the long run, we must spend time determining what the top priority is and protect it at all costs through the most powerful word in the English language: "No."

That brings us to the second point. Everything in life is a choice. It is a choice to do the online modules, to get your charts signed before you leave work that day. Yet, most doctors think that their choices are not their own. They have given their autonomy to their employer, boss, or group. Only when physicians realize their power and self-worth can they begin to stand up and require the change that is needed in their lives.

When we say "yes" to anything and everything at work, we are also saying "no" to what matters most. Fortunately, the opposite is also true. When we say "no" to anything that is not a priority to us, we are saying "Hell Yes" to things that matter most. This is when your schedule will finally begin to reflect your priorities, but it will not happen by accident.

## HELL YES POLICY

There is a well-known parable that was circulated online in the 2000s.[40] It goes like this:

There once was a philosophy professor who was giving a lecture. In front of him, he had a big glass jar, a pile of rocks, a bag of small pebbles, a tub of sand, and a bottle of water.

He started off by filling up the jar with the big rocks, and when they reached the rim of the jar, he held it up to the students and asked them if the jar was full. They all agreed there was no more room; it was full.

"Is it full?" he asked.

He then picked up the bag of small pebbles and poured them in

---

40  Try as I might, I cannot find the original source of this parable. If you do, let me know and it'll make its way into this book! This current iteration was found here: https://www.clairenewton.co.za/my-articles/the-rocks-pebbles-and-sand-story.html.

the jar. He shook the jar so that the pebbles filled the space around the big rocks. "Is the jar full now?" he asked. The group of students all looked at each other and agreed that the jar was now completely full.

"Is it really full?" he asked.

The professor then picked up the tub of sand. He poured the sand in between the pebbles and the rocks, and once again he held up the jar to his class and asked if it was full. Once again the students agreed that the jar was full.

"Are you sure it's full?" he asked.

He finally picked up a bottle of water and tipped the water into the jar until it soaked up all of the remaining space in the sand. The students laughed.

The professor went on to explain that the jar of rocks, pebbles, sand, and water represents everything that is in one's life.

This parable is powerful, because it proves the importance of knowing your priorities in life. If we put the large rocks in first, then the pebbles, and finally the sand and water—we can squeeze it all in. However, if we filled the container up with water first and then tried adding the sand, pebbles, and large rocks...well we would end up with a huge mess, wouldn't we? This is exactly how life works, too.

## PRIORITIES EXERCISE

Let's go through a short exercise to illustrate this point.

First, I want you to take out a piece of paper. Then, I want you to list your top ten priorities in order of their importance. No more, and no less. Try to be as specific as possible. For example, if you are married with children, you cannot write down "family" as one of your priorities. You need to write down "marriage" and "kids" separately because we all know that a date night alone with your spouse produces a very different result than playing a board game at the table as a family. Both are important, but over a period of five years, all board games and no date nights may not produce the results you want in the long run.

All right, it is your turn. Take some time. Hit pause. Whip out that pen and paper. If you can't find any, you can also use the space I've provided below to make your list. Then, list out your top ten priorities.

1.

2.

3.

4.

5.

6.

7.

8.

9.

10.

After you have completed your list, I want you to look it over. Can you be more specific? If so, give it a try, but you still only get to keep ten top priorities. If you wrote down family and then separated it into marriage and kids, then you need to kick out something else in order to make more room for your top ten.

After you have done this, I want you to remember what McKeown taught us about priorities. When you have a bunch of priorities, it really means that you don't have a top priority at all. So, we are going to channel our inner McKeown by taking our top ten list and whittling it down to a list of your top five priorities. You heard that right. You have to take your list of ten and make it five. Take a moment, and do that now.

1.

2.

3.

4.

5.

This exercise proves challenging, doesn't it? If you glossed over it, stop. Do not pass Go. Do not collect $200. Hit pause and go get the pen. This is important work. Don't worry; I'll wait while you do it.

This exercise was (and continues to be) a challenge for me. When my initial list included things like my marriage, kids, faith, best friends, health, clinical research, patient care, educating residents, writing my new book, clients, the two podcasts I host each week, so on and so forth...and I only got to pick ten, it was hard. Getting down to five? That feels impossible, doesn't it? How do we go about choosing? What if I asked you to whittle it down further into a top-three list? Or perhaps even a number one overall priority as the word was originally intended in the 1400s when it was created?

The point here is that we often tell ourselves that we have more priorities than it would ever be possible to maintain. When this happens, we do what most people do—we try to fit everything in and then find we are surprised when we don't have time for some of the things that matter most on paper. When we are constantly putting all of the grease on the squeaky wheel, we ignore things that don't make noise at all until they break. This often includes our relationships, health, and mental well-being.

How do you prevent this from happening? The answer is that you reverse this process. Instead of letting your schedule dictate what happens in life, you set very intentional priorities and make sure that your schedule reflects that list. This is one of the ways that you can reclaim your personal and professional autonomy to create the work-life balance we all want.

By placing our priorities onto our schedule in the proper order, we are able to fit in everything that matters to us. However, this requires us to put the big rocks in the jar of life first. These big rocks in our lives form what I call your "Hell Yes Policy." The "Hell Yes Policy" is a promise to schedule first things first and to say no to anything that does not make you say "Hell Yes!" In other words, if something isn't a top priority to you, then you say no so that you don't waste your most precious commodity (i.e., time) on anything that isn't a top priority for you. This is how you avoid putting the water into the jar first and then causing a big splash when you try to add the big rocks later. When we continually say no to the big rocks in our life, we risk waking up five or ten years from now having lived a life where we kept delaying the things that matter most because we would get to them "someday" when we had time. Only to find that it never happened.

In anesthesiology, we prevent catastrophic mistakes by asking two questions when it comes to risk/benefit conversations regarding patient care. The first question is to consider how likely a bad outcome is to happen. If it is highly unlikely, and benefits exist, then this school of thought would tell you that it is reasonable to proceed. For example, we know that for every 250,000 spinal anesthetics that we place, there will be one patient who will have an epidural hematoma that may necessitate neurosurgical decompression due to neurologic compromise. To put this in perspective, according to the CDC, the risk of getting struck by lightning is approximately one in 500,000.[41] In other words, the risk of an epidural hematoma is pretty low, and since it provides the benefit of allowing a mom-to-be to undergo a C-section without having to miss the birth of her child or allows an elderly and ill patient to avoid general anesthesia and intubation, we are willing to take this risk.

However, we must ask a second question when it comes to a risk/benefit analysis, which places its focus less on the likelihood that something bad will happen and, instead, focuses squarely on how devastating that potential bad outcome would be if it does hap-

---

41 "Lightning: Victim Data," Centers for Disease Control and Prevention, last reviewed December 23, 2013, https://www.cdc.gov/disasters/lightning/victimdata.html.

pen. Getting struck by lightning, for example, can prove fatal. For this reason, we will not take the risk of walking outside during a lightning storm unless the potential benefit outweighs the rare but deadly risk, should it happen. The same is said in the aforementioned example of an epidural hematoma. When a patient has an epidural hematoma, the impact can be devastating, including permanent paralysis if it is not diagnosed and decompressed by a spine surgeon within hours. This is why we do not perform spinal anesthetics on patients taking anticoagulants unless they've stopped the medication in enough time to allow it to wash out of their system.

It works the same way with our schedules. When we say yes to something that isn't on our Hell Yes Policy, what will be the downstream consequence to our priorities? Let's ask the same questions we ask in medicine about the risk to your priorities: if you say yes to a low-priority item, how likely is it that this will lead to a negative consequence? And how devastating will that consequence be if you continue to say yes to things that aren't your top priority?

The answer is that when our schedule is continually full of low-priority items, the chance that a negative outcome will occur is extremely high. For example, when you are approached to write the book chapter, help with the committee, provide the presentation, complete that one online module, or pick up that extra shift—these all might seem innocuous. However, with each individual task you add to your schedule, something else must give. When you say yes to one thing, you are really saying no to what matters most. You are putting the water and sand in the jar before the big rocks in your life. It is a death by a thousand paper cuts. What will your life look like five, ten, or twenty years from now when you constantly say no to things like eight hours of sleep, exercise, date nights with your partner, and time with your kids?

The likelihood that this negatively impacts your top priorities is not only high, but the results are likely to be devastating. It is a double whammy, and social science backs this up as well. Studies have shown that children who spend more quality time with their parents are more likely to have less behavioral problems in school. They experience lower rates of alcohol and drug use and are more likely to be physically active.[42] Maybe this is why the motivational speaker Zig Ziglar so wisely said, "To a child, love is spelled T-I-M-E." Quality time cannot be replaced with expensive toys and gadgets. We aren't going to buy ourselves out of not spending time with our kids. They don't want our money. And as awesome as we are, our kids do not want our abilities or talents either. They want our availability. And the consequences of not spending regular quality time with kids can prove devastating.

Hopefully, by this point I've proven to you the necessity of putting first things first. So, let's go back to that list of top-five priorities that will form your Hell Yes Policy, and then let's intentionally place those items into your schedule so that you can harness the autonomy of the self-determined physician.

My top-five list consists of my marriage, children, health, clinical work, and writing this book right now. Like the big rocks in the philosophical jar, these things go on the calendar first. I spend time blocking out date nights with Kristen. Then, I'll put family time on the calendar, like going to church on Sunday or our family movie or board game nights on Fridays. Then, I make time for exercise because I know that working out three to five times each week will not happen by accident. Finally, I block out time to write this book.

If I have time for other demands, I might say yes, but only once the big rocks in my Hell Yes Policy have been placed. If I can't, then I will simply say no. This is what resulted in me saying no to producing podcasts while I wrote this book for ten weeks. This isn't to say that

---

42  Catherine Jones, "What Are the Benefits of Spending Quality Time with Your Kids," 10 Minutes of Quality Time (website), 2017, https://10minutesof qualitytime.com/what-are-the-benefits-spending-quality-time-kids/.

other things aren't important to me. Trust me; the list of things that matter is long and extensive. However, I'll only get to those things when my Hell Yes Policy is met. Once I've made first things first. If and when those top priorities come under attack, the answer is a simple no. For example, when someone asked me to come and give a keynote speech or to consult for their institution on their culture while I was trying to write this book, the answer was typically no.

It is worth mentioning that your Hell Yes Policy will change with time. Right now I am writing this book and putting in consistent hours each week on this endeavor. This is how I've written over 60,000 words in this book in a little more than two months. When this book is done, other priorities will take its place. That may be when the keynote speeches and consulting gigs make their way back into my top priorities. Or I'll finally get Medical Degree Financial University (MDFU) off the ground to provide an online personal finance curriculum and community to physicians-in-training. It is also when the podcast episodes on *The Physician Philosopher* will come back.

Finally, it is important to mention that following a Hell Yes Policy is a constant work in progress. There will be some months where we nail it. Other weeks, we will say yes to things that put our priorities at risk. When we notice this insidious creep, we can note it and then make a change. Scheduling your priorities is an iterative process. As we discussed in a previous chapter, shoulding ourselves into shame isn't the answer. You are learning. To this day, I continue to learn alongside you! When you fail to put first things first, choose curiosity over shame and figure out how to create the life you love.

If Bill Gates needed to place big rocks into his calendar in order to make time for his "think weeks," the odds are that we need to intentionally place the big rocks of our Hell Yes Policy into our calendars, too. When we do this, it requires us to learn how to say no to anything that does not make us say Hell Yes. With practice, this is a skill we can cultivate. Once we do, personal and professional autonomy becomes much more attainable. One of the quickest ways to learn this skill is through harnessing the power of thought work, but in order to do this, we have to avoid the most common mistake I see doctors make—trying to do this work on their own.

# The Therapeutic Window of Thought Work

"When a person's down in the world, I think an ounce
of help is better than a pound of preaching."
—Edward Bulwer-Lytton

JOHN WOODEN IS widely considered the greatest coach of all time
in any sport. When Wooden took over at UCLA in the 1940s, it was a
little-known basketball program. Yet, by the time Wooden finished
his tenure, UCLA had won ten national championships, including a
stretch from 1966 until 1973 when UCLA won seven straight. In the
same time span, UCLA was 204-6. They only lost six games in seven
years. Wooden's overall record during his tenure at UCLA includes
620 wins to only 147 losses. No matter how you look at Wooden's
coaching resumé, it is easy to see why he is considered the greatest
of all time (GOAT).

It is widely said that Wooden rarely spoke about winning and instead focused on effort. Wooden famously said, "Success comes from knowing that you did your best to become the best that you are capable of becoming." You'll note that this definition of success doesn't mention winning championships, rings, or even individual games. Success is knowing that you did your best and worked to your potential. This may remind you of the concepts we discussed earlier about the journey being more important than the destination.

Wooden was a master of mindset. He demanded that his players try their best, and if he felt that they weren't living up to their potential, he would cancel the practice. Wooden felt that tiny details led to big results. This explains why he not only told his players how to play basketball but also spent time teaching them how to put on their socks in order to prevent blisters. Wooden taught his players that when you take care of the small things, the big things become easy.

Yet, my favorite teaching from John Wooden is his focus on inner work. Wooden said, "The best competition I have is against myself to become better." With an internal focus, he cared very little about comparing himself to others. He encouraged his players to do the same. Instead of focusing on an opponent, Wooden was famous for encouraging his players to focus on their own game. He was well known for rarely studying his opponents. Instead, his players spent their time and energy working on becoming the best version of themselves. This focus on the process is what allowed Wooden and his teams at UCLA to win ten NCAA championships by the end of his tenure. A record number of wins that is likely to never be toppled.

## BECOME SELF-DETERMINED

What can we learn from Wooden? It is possible to become self-determined even if the medical system does its best to try and prevent that. In Parts 1 and 2 of this book, I discussed a lot of the systemic and individual problems that plague physicians. I touched on arrival fallacies, victim mindsets, burnout, and learned helplessness, and I briefly introduced imposter syndrome. Then, I introduced you to the ABCs (autonomy, belonging, and competence) of self-determined physicians.

Unfortunately, most of us recognize that while this all sounds well and good, many institutions where we work refuse to change the focus of their current profit-over-people model. This is what produces the systemic moral injury that exists in medicine that is hell-bent on burning physicians out. This systemic problem is our "opponent."

There is a two-part mission here. The first is to fix the systematic issues that plague medicine. The second is to realize that—instead of focusing on our opponent—we can choose to focus on our own game. Like Wooden, we can learn to become the hero of our own story by focusing internally and refusing to focus on the game being played by administrators, insurance companies, and other stakeholders. We can harness the power of our mindset, money, and time to achieve our own victory over the system, instead of letting the system beat us.

Parts 3 and 4 were then meant to help you learn how to play that game. To empower you to create a life you love, even if you are working in an institution that is reluctant to change its ways and to adopt a people-first focus. Yet, if I left you here, our work would not be complete. While you can do this work on your own, you don't have to do it by yourself.

## THE BENEFITS OF COACHING

Whether someone is winning NCAA championships, learning how to practice medicine, or working toward defeating burnout and creating self-determination, having someone show us the way and help us focus on the process is key. While you can do much of the work described in this book on your own, it is important to realize that you don't *have* to do it on your own. Coaching, whether in basketball, golf, racing, acting, singing, or life, all works the same way. Coaches serve as a mirror for your current situation.

We have established the cost of burnout on medicine. We mentioned the work done by the American College of Physicians in 2019 that attributed approximately $5 BILLION in costs in the United States healthcare system to burnout.[43] This led to a 2019 *JAMA Internal Medicine* article out of the Mayo Clinic.[44] Dr. Dyrbye's team set out to answer the question of whether professional coaching helps burned-out physicians. They took eighty-eight internal medicine, pediatric, and family medicine physicians and randomized them into one of two groups. The intervention group received six coaching sessions from a professional coach via telephone. The first was for an hour, and the following five were for thirty minutes. So, they received a total of 3.5 hours of professional coaching. This occurred over a five-month period.

Now, you might argue that the reason that coaching worked for the intervention group is that they had less work during the time that they received coaching. They didn't have to see the same number of patients, right? Not to fear, the team running the study was wise in recognizing this would be a confounding variable in the study. So, all of the doctors in the coaching group were required to make up any patient volume they missed while getting coached. In other words, coaching *added* to their already busy schedule.

They compared this to the control group who did not receive

---

43   Han et al., "Physician Burnout," *Annals of Internal Medicine*, June 4, 2019, https://doi.org/10.7326/M18-1422.

44   Dyrbye et al., "Effect of a Professional Coaching Intervention," *JAMA Internal Medicine*, https://doi.org/10.1001/jamainternmed.2019.2425.

professional coaching. The results from this study showed that physicians who received 3.5 hours of coaching over five months had 30% less emotional exhaustion compared to the control group. They also showed a 20% decrease in burnout and improved quality of life and resilience. Simply put, professional coaching for physicians works. This is despite adding the coaching on top of their work, which you could argue should have made these metrics worse and not better. Coaching helps physicians to reclaim a sense of professional and personal autonomy that they currently lack while experiencing burnout from the institutions that morally injure them. The Cleveland Clinic experienced the power of coaching, too, when they estimated that the hospital saved $133 million due to physician coaching as it led to lower turnover rates among their doctors.

Coaching helps doctors improve their personal and professional autonomy. It also helps doctors improve the perception of their accomplishments. Yet, there is a third reason that coaching helps burned-out doctors. Many coaching programs include group coaching experiences that foster a deep and meaningful sense of community, where burned-out physicians can feel that they belong. When doctors see other physicians who are going through the same shared and lived experiences, there is a very deep and meaningful connection, a sense that they are a member of the same team. This is why literature has shown the benefit of shared peer-to-peer interactions in burned-out physicians.

Remember, the belonging that self-determined physicians require is composed of two parts. The first is to feel like a valued member of a team, which group coaching often provides. The second component of belonging is feeling attached to a deeper purpose, and physician coaching allows doctors to band together on the same team. A team working to end the morally injurious culture that exists in medicine. In other words, coaching helps physicians master all of the ABCs of self-determination—autonomy, belonging, and their perceived competence. It helps them create personal and professional autonomy in their life, fosters belonging through shared experiences and being connected to a deeper purpose of improving the culture of medicine, and improves their real and perceived competence.

Yet as I mentioned earlier, the most common mistake that I see doctors make is thinking that they are alone on this journey. They rail against the system that refuses to change, read self-help books to find some sense of solace, work on their thought work and gratitude, and end up feeling just as burned out as they ever were.

## COACHING FOR PHYSICIANS BY PHYSICIANS

The best aspect of thought work for physicians is that doctors suddenly realize that while the medical system is completely and utterly broken, they don't have to wait for that system to change in order to have some reprieve from their suffering. This is the power that allows physicians to reclaim their personal and professional autonomy. It can also help them defeat their imposter syndrome. There is hope on the horizon. Light at the end of what was previously a pitch-black tunnel. They start to see that while they used to feel trapped in medicine and completely powerless in their situation, they have more power than they ever realized. Doctors who put the hours into honing these skills transition from being the victim of their story to finally becoming the hero. That is why I wrote this book.

My hope is that this book serves as a primer or foundation for you to start your work toward becoming like Nelson Mandela, Rosa Parks, and Rubin "Hurricane" Carter. I hope it allows you to take away very real and tangible ways to improve your life. If you stop there, congratulations! You have still accomplished far more than the vast majority of doctors out there who aren't even aware of this work (yet)!

However, for those of you who realize that coaching can serve as a catalyst to help you get to your goals faster, I want to let you know how to find a coach or coaching program that would work for you. While there are many great coaching programs out there, not all of them are created equal. So, if you decide that you don't want to do it all by yourself, then I highly encourage you to consider finding a coach that fits your needs.

When looking for a coach, it is also crucial to find someone who resonates with you. If you want to become a professional golfer, for example, it would probably be helpful to work with a golf pro. Not a singing coach. Similarly, if you are trying to build a business, working with someone who is an entrepreneur is helpful. It is the same with physician coaching. Finding someone who has walked in your shoes, who can come alongside you and ask questions that provide insight into your situation, can make all the difference. This is one reason that I do not receive life coaching from other professional coaches who are not physicians. I want to spend time getting coached, not explaining what an FTE, EMR, or Level 1 trauma is to the person coaching me. I also want a coach who has successfully helped others transition from where I am to where I want to be.

Finally, and most importantly, when looking for a coach, we have discussed the importance of causal coaching. While there is an endless list of people out there who are willing to tell you what to do or how to do it without making a proper diagnosis first, determining what the problem is *first* is vital for success. Causal coaching makes the diagnosis. While many clients come into coaching expecting to be told what to do to fix their problems, that is not the solution to their struggles. You are a highly intelligent, hardworking, and educated physician. As a coach, who am I to presume that I know better than you what is best for your life? If I simply told our physician clients to meditate more, eat well and exercise, practice good sleep hygiene, and go part-time...do you think this would solve their problems? No. That is treating the symptoms instead of the disease.

This is why "good" coaching is synonymous with causal coaching, or the kind of coaching where the coach helps you determine the root thoughts that are *causing* your feelings, actions, and how you show up in this world. Causal coaching is the work of helping the person make the diagnosis, instead of treating the symptoms by slapping a Band-Aid on it. Not every coach follows a causal coaching model. So, make sure that they are more focused on making the diagnosis than they are on telling you what to do.

## HOW TO CONTINUE YOUR JOURNEY

After making it this far in this book, you might ask why I am "giving the milk away" for less than $30. First, and most importantly, I genuinely enjoy helping people. I am one of those crazy people who believes that doctors can still change medicine. Only when we have enough physicians who are empowered to stand up will our broken medical system be required to change. Ultimately, that is the real purpose behind everything we do at The Physician Philosopher— creating a team of like-minded physicians who can band together to fix this mess called medicine. The more doctors we have on this journey heading toward self-determination, the better.

For those who are sick and tired of being sick and tired, I don't promise you that the work will be easy, but I do promise you it will be worth it. As the Albert Einstein quote at the beginning of this book reminds us, *"We can't solve problems by using the same kind of thinking we used when we created them."* As you start the next step of your journey, wherever that may lead, I hope this book has changed your thinking. I hope it has encouraged you to embrace failure, self-compassion, thought work, and to learn how to enjoy the journey along the way. And while you can do it on your own, know that you do not have to. Don't wait for the perfect time to get going. Instead, start before you're ready. Start by starting. Start now.

# ACKNOWLEDGMENTS

THIS BOOK TOOK approximately a year to write, edit, and publish. Honestly, the reason that it didn't take longer is because of the amazing team and support that I have around me. So, I would be remiss if I failed to mention the people who made this book possible.

Kristen, you are and have always been my much better half. You keep me centered and pull me back to the cross when I run astray. Without your grace, forgiveness, and understanding this book would not have been possible. Thank you for being my rock, particularly in the times when my depression leaves me a shell of myself. You never give up on me. I don't deserve you, but I thank God for you each and every day—even on the days I forget to tell you. I love you.

Grace, Wesley, and Anna Ruth. Thank you for the many stories, some of which even graced the pages of this book. Never forget, I love each of you more than I could ever say. Through my mistakes, I hope that you have seen what grace, forgiveness, and self-compassion look like. Thanks for loving your very imperfect dad. I would move mountains for each of you. You are my world.

Kristin, you make everything at The Physician Philosopher work. You are the secret sauce. I hope you know that I will never forget that. Thank you for being our amazing business manager and, more importantly, for being the best big sister a little brother could ask for. I've enjoyed nothing more in this business than the opportunity to grow in a deeper relationship with you. I love you. (PS, Lance, I see you! Thank you for letting me borrow your bride so often! I owe you a beer or two the next time I am in Seattle. And I probably owe you another every other time after that, too.)

To my "Framily," thank you for being there. While you may not always understand the crazy world that is my brain, you are willing to listen to my passionate tirades about how things are and how they could be better. You are always there in real life when I need you—including when my depression rears its ugly head and threatens all that is good in our world. Thanks for loving me and supporting me.

Dr. Tricia James—what a friend (and coach) you are to me. Not only were you an amazing coach to me while writing this book—*yes, Dr. Tricia James is my coach; you should go and look her up*! Tricia, you held space for my crazy brain that has a tendency to act like a tangential toddler on steroids. You were one of the only people who I gave the ugly first draft of this book to who read it, provided thoughts, and were all in on this book from the beginning. You are awesome. I'm here for you if and when you ever need it.

I'd also like to extend a special thanks to the anesthesiology department at Wake Forest where I worked as I wrote this book. Specifically, I'd like to thank Dr. Randy Calicott. Thank you for investing in me by both reading this book and fighting for me to have a predictable schedule so that I had the time off to dedicate to it. (PS, Randy, thanks for being a constant sounding board from which much of this book sprang to life.)

When it came to getting help editing and publishing this book, I used SCRIBE Media to take the reins of this project. You all made what I think was an already pretty good book into an amazing one that is going to change the landscape of medicine. You heard it here first, but I couldn't have done it without SCRIBE's help.

Specifically, at SCRIBE Media, I'd like to thank Eliece Pool, my publication manager who ran the show from the beginning. Thank you for keeping me organized! Nicole Jobe, Tara Taylor, and Josh

Rahn, you made editing this book fun and you improved the book from the jump. Thank you for your ideas, and for pointing out when mine had gone astray! Chelsea McGuckin—what a rock star! Your very first cover design was the one to keep. Thank you for taking my vision and making it a reality. Of course, I'd like to thank all of the remaining editors and those running things behind the scenes!

Finally, I'd like to thank all of the coaches and clients inside of ACE. I love our community and am constantly blown away that I get to hang out with you each week. This work matters. You are the reason I show up every day in this business!

That's it, folks! Until next time ... Start before you're ready! Start by starting! Start now!

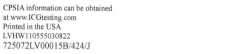